Central Sleep Apnea

Editor

PETER C. GAY

SLEEP MEDICINE CLINICS

www.sleep.theclinics.com

Consulting Editor
TEOFILO LEE-CHIONG Jr

March 2014 • Volume 9 • Number 1

ELSEVIER

1600 John F. Kennedy Boulevard • Suite 1800 • Philadelphia, Pennsylvania, 19103-2899

http://www.theclinics.com

SLEEP MEDICINE CLINICS Volume 9, Number 1
March 2014, ISSN 1556-407X, ISBN-13: 978-0-323-28722-7

Editor: Patrick Manley
Developmental Editor: Donald Mumford

Sleep Medicine Clinics (ISSN 1556-407X) is published quarterly by Elsevier Inc., 360 Park Avenue South, New York, NY 10010-1710. Months of issue are March, June, September and December. Business and Editorial Offices: 1600 John F. Kennedy Blvd., Ste. 1800, Philadelphia, PA 19103-2899. Customer Service Office: 3251 Riverport Lane, Maryland Heights, MO 63043. Periodicals postage paid at New York, NY and additional mailing offices. Subscription prices are $195.00 per year (US individuals), $95.00 (US residents), $406.00 (US institutions), $230.00 (Canadian individuals), $235.00 (foreign individuals), $135.00 (Canadian and foreign residents) and $452.00 (Canadian and foreign institutions). Foreign air speed delivery is included in all Clinics subscription prices. All prices are subject to change without notice. **POSTMASTER:** Send change of address to Sleep Medicine Clinics, Elsevier Health Sciences Division, Subscription Customer Service, 3251 Riverport Lane, Maryland Heights, MO 63043. Customer Service: **Tel: 1-800-654-2452 (U.S. and Canada); 314-447-8871 (outside U.S. and Canada). Fax: 314-447-8029. E-mail: journalscustomerservice-usa@elsevier.com (for print support); journalsonlinesupport-usa@elsevier.com (for online support).**

Reprints. For copies of 100 or more of articles in this publication, please contact the Commercial Reprints Department, Elsevier Inc., 360 Park Avenue South, New York, NY 10010-1710. Tel.: 212-633-3874; Fax: 212-633-3820; E-mail: reprints@elsevier.com.

Printed and bound by CPI Group (UK) Ltd, Croydon, CR0 4YY

PROGRAM OBJECTIVE

The goal of *Sleep Clinics of North America* is to keep practicing physicians up to date with current clinical practice by providing timely articles reviewing the state of the art in patient care.

TARGET AUDIENCE

All practicing physicians and other healthcare professionals.

LEARNING OBJECTIVES

Upon completion of this activity, participants will be able to:
1. Discuss central hyperventilation syndromes.
2. Identify central sleep apnea due to other medical disorders.
3. Describe alternative approaches to treatment of central sleep apnea.

ACCREDITATION

The Elsevier Office of Continuing Medical Education (EOCME) is accredited by the Accreditation Council for Continuing Medical Education (ACCME) to provide continuing medical education for physicians.

The EOCME designates this enduring material for a maximum of 15 *AMA PRA Category 1 Credit*(s)™. Physicians should claim only the credit commensurate with the extent of their participation in the activity.

All other health care professionals requesting continuing education credit for this enduring material will be issued a certificate of participation.

DISCLOSURE OF CONFLICTS OF INTEREST

The EOCME assesses conflict of interest with its instructors, faculty, planners, and other individuals who are in a position to control the content of CME activities. All relevant conflicts of interest that are identified are thoroughly vetted by EOCME for fair balance, scientific objectivity, and patient care recommendations. EOCME is committed to providing its learners with CME activities that promote improvements or quality in healthcare and not a specific proprietary business or a commercial interest.

The planning committee, staff, authors and editors listed below have identified no financial relationships or relationships to products or devices they or their spouse/life partner have with commercial interest related to the content of this CME activity:
Sean M. Caples, DO; Christopher M. Cielo, DO; Sally L. Davidson Ward, MD; Danny Joel Eckert, PhD; Peter C. Gay, MD, MS; Kristen Helm; Brynne Hunter; Mithri R. Junna, MD; Salman Raza Khan, MD; Bhanu Prakash Kolla, MD, MRCPsych; Sandy Lavery; Patrick Manley, Meghna P. Mansukhani, MD; Rodrigo Tomazini Martins, MD; Jill McNair; Timothy I. Morgenthaler, MD; Mahalakshmi Narayanan; Kannan Ramar, MD; Bernardo J. Selim, MD.

The planning committee, staff, authors and editors listed below have identified financial relationships or relationships to products or devices they or their spouse/life partner have with commercial interest related to the content of this CME activity:
Teofilo Lee-Chiong Jr, MD is a consultant/advisor for CareCore National and Elsevier; has employment affiliation, has stock ownership in, and receives a research grant from Phillips Respironics; has royalties/patents with Elsevier.
Shahrokh Javaheri, MD is on speakers bureau for Philips Respironics and ResMed; has a research grant from Philips Respironics; and is a consultant/advisor for Respicardia, Inc.
Carole L. Marcus, MBBCh has a research grant with Philips Respironics; has royalties/patents with Elsevier.
Matthew T. Naughton, MBBS, MD, FRACP has a research grant ResMed.
Winfried J. Randerath, MD; has research grants with, is a consultant/advisor and is on speakers bureau for Weinmann Medical Technology GmBH & Co., Philips Respironics and ResMed.
Robert Joseph Thomas, MD, MMSc has research grants with DeVilbiss Healthcare LLC and Gerson Lehrman Group, Inc; has patent for a device to treat central /complex apnea with carbon dioxide; has patent for ECG-based software to phenotype sleep and sleep apnea, licensed to MyCardio, LLC.

UNAPPROVED/OFF-LABEL USE DISCLOSURE

The EOCME requires CME faculty to disclose to the participants:
1. When products or procedures being discussed are off-label, unlabelled, experimental, and/or investigational (not US Food and Drug Administration (FDA) approved); and
2. Any limitations on the information presented, such as data that are preliminary or that represent ongoing research, interim analyses, and/or unsupported opinions. Faculty may discuss information about pharmaceutical agents that is outside of FDA-approved labelling. This information is intended solely for CME and is not intended to promote off-label use of these medications. If you have any questions, contact the medical affairs department of the manufacturer for the most recent prescribing information.

TO ENROLL

To enroll in the Sleep Medicines Clinic Continuing Medical Education program, call customer service at 1-800-654-2452 or sign up online at http://www.theclinics.com/home/cme. The CME program is available to subscribers for an additional annual fee of USD $126.

METHOD OF PARTICIPATION

In order to claim credit, participants must complete the following:
1. Complete enrolment as indicated above.
2. Read the activity.
3. Complete the CME Test and Evaluation. Participants must achieve a score of 70% on the test. All CME Tests and Evaluations must be completed online.

CME INQUIRIES/SPECIAL NEEDS

For all CME inquiries or special needs, please contact elsevierCME@elsevier.com.

SLEEP MEDICINE CLINICS

FORTHCOMING ISSUES

June 2014
Behavioral Aspects of Sleep Problems in Childhood and Adolescence
Judith Owens, *Editor*

September 2014
Evaluation of Sleep Complaints
Clete Kushida, *Editor*

December 2014
Hypoventilation Syndrome
Babak Mokhlesi, *Editor*

RECENT ISSUES

December 2013
Therapies for Obstructive Sleep Apnea
Shirley F. Jones and James A. Barker, *Editors*

September 2013
Insomnia
Jack D. Edinger, *Editor*

June 2013
Fatigue
Max Hirshkowitz and
Amir Sharafkhaneh, *Editors*

RELATED INTEREST

Clinics in Chest Medicine, September 2012 (Vol. 33, Issue 3)
Asthma
Pascal Chanez, *Editor*

Contributors

CONSULTING EDITOR

TEOFILO LEE-CHIONG Jr, MD
Professor of Medicine, Division of Pulmonary,
Critical Care and Sleep Medicine, Department
of Medicine, National Jewish Health, University
of Colorado, Denver, Colorado; Chief Medical
Liaison, Philips Respironics, Pennsylvania

EDITOR

PETER C. GAY, MD
Professor of Medicine, Mayo Clinic Rochester,
Mayo Center for Sleep Medicine, Rochester,
Minnesota

AUTHORS

SEAN M. CAPLES, DO
Assistant Professor of Medicine, Mayo Clinic
College of Medicine, Division of Pulmonary and
Critical Care Medicine, Center for Sleep
Medicine, Mayo Clinic, Rochester, Minnesota

CHRISTOPHER M. CIELO, DO
Fellow, Sleep Medicine and Pulmonary
Medicine, Division of Pulmonary Medicine,
The Children's Hospital of Philadelphia,
Philadelphia, Pennsylvania

SALLY L. DAVIDSON WARD, MD
Division of Pediatric Pulmonology,
Children's Hospital Los Angeles, Los Angeles,
California

DANNY JOEL ECKERT, PhD
Neuroscience Research Australia (NeuRA),
School of Medical Sciences, University of
New South Wales, Randwick, Sydney,
New South Wales, Australia

SHAHROKH JAVAHERI, MD
Emeritus Professor of Medicine, University of
Cincinnati, College of Medicine, Cincinnati;
Medical Director, Sleepcare Diagnostics,
Mason, Ohio

MITHRI R. JUNNA, MD
Department of Neurology, Assistant
Professor in Neurology, Mayo Clinic Center
for Sleep Medicine, Mayo Clinic, Rochester,
Minnesota

SALMAN RAZA KHAN, MD
Division of Pediatric Pulmonology, Children's
Hospital Los Angeles, Los Angeles, California

BHANU PRAKASH KOLLA, MD, MRCPsych
Consultant Physician, Psychiatry and Sleep
Medicine, Affiliated Communities Medical
Center, Willmar, Minnesota

MEGHNA P. MANSUKHANI, MD
Consultant Physician, Sleep Medicine,
Affiliated Communities Medical Center,
Willmar, Minnesota

CAROLE L. MARCUS, MBBCh
Director, Department of Pediatrics, Sleep
Center, The Children's Hospital of Philadelphia,
Professor of Pediatrics, The University of
Pennsylvania Perelman School of Medicine,
Philadelphia, Pennsylvania

RODRIGO TOMAZINI MARTINS, MD
Neurology Department, Instituto de
Neurologia de Curitiba, Ecoville, Curitiba,
Parana, Brazil; Neuroscience Research
Australia (NeuRA), School of Medical Sciences,
University of New South Wales, Randwick,
Sydney, New South Wales, Australia

TIMOTHY I. MORGENTHALER, MD
Division of Pulmonary and Critical Care
Medicine, Patient Safety Officer, Professor
of Medicine, Mayo Clinic Center for Sleep
Medicine, Mayo Clinic, Rochester, Minnesota

**MATTHEW T. NAUGHTON, MBBS, MD,
FRACP**
Head, General Respiratory and Sleep Medicine,
Department of Allergy, Immunology and
Respiratory Medicine, Alfred Hospital, Monash
University, Melbourne, Victoria, Australia

KANNAN RAMAR, MD
Consultant Physician, Division of Pulmonary
and Critical Care Medicine, Center for Sleep
Medicine, Associate Professor of Medicine,
Mayo College of Medicine, Mayo Clinic,
Rochester, Minnesota

WINFRIED J. RANDERATH, MD, FCCP
Professor of Medicine, Institute of
Pneumology, University Witten/Herdecke,
Clinic for Pneumology and Allergology, Center
of Sleep Medicine and Respiratory Care,
Bethanien Hospital, Solingen, Germany

BERNARDO J. SELIM, MD
Division of Pulmonary and Critical Care
Medicine, Assistant Professor in Medicine,
Mayo Clinic Center for Sleep Medicine, Mayo
Clinic, Rochester, Minnesota

ROBERT JOSEPH THOMAS, MD, MMSc
Division of Pulmonary, Critical Care and Sleep,
Department of Medicine, Beth Israel
Deaconess Medical Center, Associate
Professor of Medicine, Harvard Medical
School, Boston, Massachusetts

Contents

This review summarizes the main features of the different central sleep apnea syndromes (CSASs) based on the International Classification of Sleep Disorders, 2nd edition, and provides a management overview of the different CSASs in the adult population based on the current recommendations from the American Academy of Sleep Medicine practice parameters.

Cheyne-Stokes respiration with central sleep apnea (CSA-CSR) is a disorder commonly seen in patients with heart failure and characterized by cyclic hyperventilation with hypocapnia, which distinguishes it from obstructive sleep apnea and disorders of hypoventilation. The response of CSA-CSR to therapies targeted at the failing heart is proportional to the improvement in cardiac function. The apnea-hypopnea index is a crude marker of CSA-CSR severity and consideration should always be given to collateral history and examination, plus markers of cardiac and sleep dysfunction, plus quality of life when deciding to monitor or manage.

Central sleep apnea (CSA) syndromes have been studied extensively in the setting of heart failure (HF). CSA is generally thought to occur as a consequence of HF. Some data suggest, however, that CSA may play an important role in outcomes in the HF population. For a similar degree of HF, does the presence of CSA portend a worse outcome? If so, does directed treatment of CSA impact those outcomes? The evidence to answer these questions is reviewed here. Beyond HF, the relationship between CSA and other cardiovascular diseases has been minimally explored, with the exception of atrial fibrillation.

Patients with sleep-disordered breathing exhibit abnormal patterns of breathing most often characterized by inadequate maintenance of ventilation, in the form of repetitive apneas or hypopneas, or as more sustained alveolar hypoventilation. When most repetitive abnormal events are pathophysiologically related to upper airway obstruction during adequate efforts to breathe, obstructive sleep apnea syndrome is diagnosed. In contrast, when most repetitive apneas and hypopneas result from transiently reduced efforts to breathe, central sleep apnea syndrome is diagnosed. Complex sleep apnea syndrome represents a combination of these

considered in complex apnea patients. Phenotyping of sleep apnea beyond conventional scoring approaches is the key to optimal management.

Preface
Overview of Central Sleep Apnea

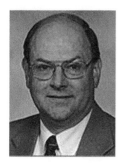

Peter C. Gay, MD
Editor

The condition of central sleep apnea (CSA) was first noted by two physicians in the 1800s. John Cheyne, from Great Britain, and William Stokes, who was schooled in Ireland, first described what later came to be known as Cheyne-Stokes Respiration.[1,2] They were more interested in heart disease and simply observed the phenomena as a cardiac problem. We have come a long way since and there are eleven articles herein that focus in some detail on a particularly pertinent set of issues regarding CSA, beginning with this overview. The reader will notice some redundancy in the articles, which were retained for emphasis and further clarity. It is hoped that a better insight into many aspects of CSA will be appreciated and new questions might be generated by our efforts.

We begin with the article, "International Classification of Sleep Disorders-2 (ICSD-2) and American Academy of Sleep Medicine (AASM) Practice Parameters," which is a summary of the main aspects of the different central sleep apnea syndromes (CSAS) as organized in the ICSD-2. This is further enhanced with a discussion of the general management of the different CSAS in adults as presented in the current recommendations from the AASM Practice Parameters.

The next article, "Cheyne-Stokes Respiration," describes CSA due to Cheyne-Stokes respiration in detail. There is thoughtful commentary on the pathophysiology and mechanisms that generate and perpetuate CSAS. A focus on the optimal treatment of the underlying heart failure is emphasized. The article, "Central Sleep Apnea and

Cardiovascular Disease" that follows extends this further to give insight into the associated CSA and cardiovascular disease, again focusing on the treatment of the underlying disorder.

We continue with reports of other forms of CSA with the now more widely recognized and accepted complex sleep apnea syndrome (Comp-SAS). The article entitled, "Complex Sleep Apnea (CompSAS)," reveals the controversy and the data supporting this disorder, why it should be considered a unique clinical problem, and how it is best treated.

With the urge to relieve pain and suffering in the medical community, there has been a surge in the use of opioids resulting in the well-known associated central apnea condition that often results. The article that investigates this disorder, "Opioids-induced Central Sleep Apnea: Mechanisms and Therapies," gives a discerning review of the sleep-disordered breathing problem that develops in these patients, which is a variant of the Comp-SAS pattern described in the previous article.

For comprehensive purposes, we added an additional article, "Central Sleep Apnea Due To Other Medical Disorders," discussing the other miscellaneous types of CSA addressing the medical disorders that provoke this, such as brain tumors, Chiari type I malformation, stroke, and a range of endocrine, hormonal, neurodegenerative, and neuromuscular diseases.

We move next to treatment methods with the mainstay treatment now being the adaptive servo-ventilator and the article, "Adaptive

Sleep Med Clin 9 (2014) xi–xii
http://dx.doi.org/10.1016/j.jsmc.2013.11.003
1556-407X/14/$ – see front matter © 2014 Elsevier Inc. All rights reserved.

Servo-Ventilation," defines the rationale and function of this device and the evidence supporting its application in these disorders. The following article, "Alternative Approaches to Treatment of Central Sleep Apnea," gives discourse regarding innovative alternatives to the treatment of resistant or intolerant patients to adaptive servo-ventilation with CSA syndromes, which also conveys a better understanding of the condition and its need for further study.

We finish with an unfamiliar topic to most clinicians caring for adult patients. They should still be aware of childhood and younger related sleep-disordered breathing problems, especially as some may grow into adulthood. The final articles, "Central Hypoventilation Syndromes in Children" and "Central Sleep Apnea in Infants," should be of particular interest for those unfamiliar with this topic or inquisitive for board review purposes.

All articles contain keyword search phrases and a synopsis for easy reading. The references are extensive and up–to-date. We accept that many busy clinicians are in need of state-of-the-art knowledge and treatment recommendations in an easily accessible way, which was the primary goal of our efforts. Enjoy.

Peter C. Gay, MD
Mayo Clinic Rochester
Mayo Center for Sleep Medicine
Rochester, MN 55905, USA

E-mail address:
pgay@mayo.ed

REFERENCES

1. Cheyne J. A case of apoplexy in which the fleshy part of the heart was converted into fat. Dublin Hospital Reports 1818;2:216–23 [Reprinted in Willius FA, Keys TE. Cardiac Classics. 1941. p. 317–320.].
2. Stokes W. Fatty degeneration of the heart. In: The diseases of the heart and aorta. Dublin: 1854. p. 320–7.

International Classification of Sleep Disorders 2 and American Academy of Sleep Medicine Practice Parameters for Central Sleep Apnea

Meghna P. Mansukhani, MD[a],
Bhanu Prakash Kolla, MD, MRCPsych[b], Kannan Ramar, MD[c],*

KEYWORDS

- Central sleep apnea • Cheyne-Stokes breathing pattern • Congestive heart failure
- Periodic breathing • Sleep apnea of infancy • Adaptive servoventilator

KEY POINTS

- Though central sleep apnea syndromes are treated with positive airway pressure therapies, further long-term studies are required to address the effects on hospital admission rates, morbidity, and mortality.
- Additional studies comparing the relative cost-effectiveness, risks, and benefits of various treatment modalities are needed.
- More research on multimodality titration polysomnograms that use a different device when the previous one seems to be unsuccessful may eventually help reduce testing time and health care costs.

INTRODUCTION

Sleep disorders are classified into 8 main categories based on the International Classification of Sleep Disorders, Second Edition (ICSD-2).[1] The ICSD-2 helps provide a consistent framework for clinicians and researchers to categorize and define sleep and arousal disorders in a structured, scientific, rational, and practical manner. It is compatible with the International Classification of Diseases, Tenth Revision (ICD-10). Central sleep apnea syndromes (CSASs) are in the category of sleep-related breathing disorders (SRBDs) and are characterized by apneas with diminished or absent respiratory effort that occur in a cyclic or intermittent pattern. These apneas may be idiopathic or secondary to environmental causes, drugs, or underlying medical conditions. The various types are listed and discussed later.

The American Academy of Sleep Medicine (AASM) practice parameters are evidence-based clinical guidelines developed by the Standards of Practice Committee (SPC) for the treatment of various common sleep disorders. These parameters are approved by the Board of Directors of the AASM before publication. The practice parameters are freely accessible on the AASM Web site

Disclosures: None.
[a] Sleep Medicine, Affiliated Communities Medical Center, 101 Willmar Avenue Southwest, Willmar, MN 56201, USA; [b] Psychiatry and Sleep Medicine, Affiliated Communities Medical Center, 101 Willmar Avenue Southwest, Willmar, MN 56201, USA; [c] Division of Pulmonary and Critical Care Medicine, Center for Sleep Medicine, Mayo College of Medicine, Mayo Clinic, 200 First Street Southwest, Rochester, MN 55905, USA
* Corresponding author.
E-mail address: ramar.kannan@mayo.edu

Sleep Med Clin 9 (2014) 1–11
http://dx.doi.org/10.1016/j.jsmc.2013.10.006

and are widely used by physicians engaged in treating patients with sleep disorders, and are therefore capable of influencing not only medical decision making and patient outcomes but also health care costs.

A recent practice parameters article by Aurora and colleagues[2] discussed the treatment recommendations for CSAS in adults. The central sleep apnea (CSA) task force under the SPC conducted a PubMed search for articles from 1966 to 2010 on the medical treatment of CSAS, defined as greater than 50% central disordered breathing events including periodic breathing (if subjects presented with both CSAS and obstructive sleep apnea). Of those that met initial criteria, 77 articles were included.[2] Assessment of the quality of evidence was performed using the Grading of Recommendations Assessment, Development, and Evaluation (GRADE) process, which begins with clearly specifying the question to be answered, collecting and summarizing available data, using explicit criteria for rating the evidence, and then providing recommendations according to the strength of supporting evidence.[3] Levels of recommendations used by the AASM based on GRADE are shown in **Table 1**. All practice parameter articles published after the CSA article have used the GRADE methodology. This article summarizes the various CSASs in adults based on the ICSD-2 and the treatment options and recommendations using the practice parameters as a guide (**Box 1**).

PRIMARY CSA
Definition

As per the ICSD-2, primary CSA is characterized by at least 1 of the following: excessive daytime sleepiness, frequent arousals and awakenings during sleep, insomnia complaints, awakening short of breath, and by polysomnography (PSG) showing 5 or more central apneas per hour of sleep. The disorder is not better explained by another current sleep disorder, medical or neurologic disorder, medication use, or substance use disorder.[1]

Features

Primary CSA is idiopathic, characterized by recurrent pauses in breathing with no ventilatory effort occurring in a repetitive manner during sleep. Studies suggest that the disorder is rare, with a male predominance, and is more commonly seen in middle-aged and older individuals.[4]

Increased ventilatory response to partial pressure of carbon dioxide in blood ($Paco_2$) leading to instability in ventilatory control seems to be the predominant predisposing factor. A low normal $Paco_2$ of less than 40 mm Hg is typically seen during wakefulness in patients with this disorder. Even a small increase in ventilation in these chemosensitive individuals causes the $Paco_2$ level to decrease to less than the apnea threshold, triggering cessation in breathing.[5,6] Insomnia, nasal obstruction, and neurologic disorders with autonomic dysfunction are other reported predisposing factors.[7,8]

Central apneas are seen more commonly at sleep onset and during non–rapid eye movement (NREM) sleep than rapid eye movement (REM) sleep. These respiratory events are usually associated with only mild oxyhemoglobin desaturation. In general, patients with primary CSA do not develop pulmonary hypertension, cor pulmonale, or other adverse cardiovascular unless there is accompanying nocturnal hypoventilation with hypercapnia.

Treatment

Summary of evidence
A few small nonrandomized trials directly examining therapeutic options for primary CSA showed significant improvement in the Apnea-Hypopnea Index (AHI) with a low dose (250 mg per day) and a high dose (1000 mg per day) of acetazolamide

---

Table 1
AASM levels of recommendations

Final Standards of Practice Recommendations	Overall Quality of Evidence			
Assessment of Benefit/Harm/Burden	High	Moderate	Low	Very Low
Benefits clearly outweigh harm/burden	Standard	Standard	Guideline	Option
Benefits closely balanced with harm/burden or uncertainty in the estimates of benefit/harm/burden	Guideline	Guideline	Option	Option
Harm/burden clearly outweighs benefits	Standard	Standard	Standard	Standard

From Aurora RN, Chowdhuri S, Ramar K, et al. The treatment of central sleep apnea syndromes in adults: practice parameters with an evidence-based literature review and meta-analyses. Sleep 2012;35:21; with permission.

at 1 month and 1 week respectively.[8,9] An improvement in daytime sleepiness was noted in the low-dose group. Zolpidem showed a significant reduction in AHI along with a decrease in daytime somnolence in 20 patients at 9 weeks' follow-up,[10] although a borderline significant decrease in AHI was reported with triazolam.[11]

Carbon dioxide has been shown to decrease AHI in primary CSA[12]; however, it is not commercially available and can be difficult to titrate in an open circuit. Although there are no studies on the use of positive airway pressure (PAP) in the setting of primary CSA, it is easily available and not associated with significant adverse effects. In contrast, there is an increased risk of adverse effects with acetazolamide, zolpidem, and triazolam. In addition, zolpidem and triazolam may worsen obstructive sleep disordered breathing events and respiratory depression.

Recommendation "Positive airway pressure therapy may be considered for the treatment of primary CSAS."[2]

Level of recommendation Option.[2]

Recommendation "Acetazolamide has limited supporting evidence but may be considered for the treatment of primary CSAS."[2] Potential increased risk for adverse events should be considered.

Level of recommendation Option.[2]

Recommendation "The use of zolpidem and triazolam may be considered for the treatment of primary CSAS only if the patient does not have underlying risk factors for respiratory depression."[2] Potential increased risk for adverse events and worsening of sleep disordered breathing events should be considered.

Level of recommendation Option.[2]

CSA DUE TO CHEYNE-STOKES BREATHING PATTERN
Definition

Cheyne-Stokes breathing pattern
As per ICSD-2, Cheyne-Stokes breathing pattern (CSBP) on polysomnography is characterized by at least 10 central apneas and hypopneas per hour of sleep in which the hypopnea has a crescendo-decrescendo pattern of tidal volume accompanied by frequent arousals from sleep and derangement of sleep structure. The breathing disorder occurs in association with a serious medical illness, such as heart failure, stroke, or renal failure, and the disorder is not better explained by another current sleep disorder, medication use, or substance use disorder.[1]

Features

As with other forms of CSA, decreased central respiratory drive leads to absent or reduced ventilatory effort in a repetitive fashion, seen more commonly during NREM sleep (**Fig. 1**). Long cycle length (of more than 45 seconds) and a waxing and waning pattern differentiate CSBP from other

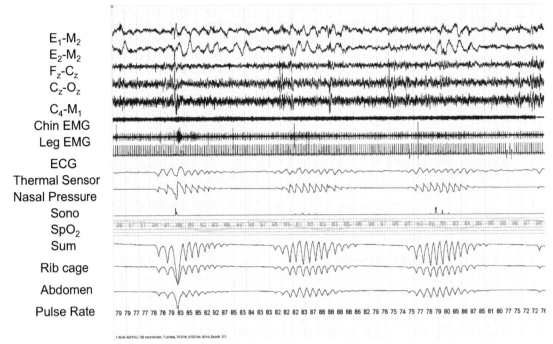

Fig. 1. CSA due to CSBP. A 180-second epoch showing a periodic breathing pattern in a patient with congestive heart failure typical for CSA caused by CSBP. ECG, electrocardiogram; EMG, electromyogram; Spo₂, oxygen saturation via pulse oximetry.

types of periodic breathing.[13] In addition, arousals generally occur a few breaths after ventilation has resumed, unlike other forms of sleep disordered breathing (SDB), in which they occur at the termination of the respiratory event.

Patients with this disorder hyperventilate chronically both during sleep and while awake, perhaps because of increased central and peripheral chemoresponsiveness, or because of stimulation of the pulmonary vagal irritant receptors by pulmonary venous congestion.[14] $Paco_2$ values tend to be in the low normal range and closer to the apnea threshold. Therefore, a small increase in minute ventilation can lead to a decrease in $Paco_2$ levels to less than the apnea threshold, resulting in central apneas.[15]

Arousals after the termination of a respiratory event cause abrupt lowering of the apnea threshold. At the same time, resumption of ventilation, and even hyperventilation, causes $Paco_2$ to decrease to less than the apnea threshold, propagating recurrent apneas.[16] $Paco_2$ changes in the lung are transmitted slowly to the chemoreceptors because of the long circulation time in congestive heart failure (CHF), resulting in a gradual crescendo-decrescendo pattern.

CSBP is more commonly seen in elderly individuals and is more common in men. Prevalence rates are 25% to 40% in patients with CHF and 10% in patients with strokes. In the setting of CHF, male gender, age more than 60 years, presence of atrial fibrillation, and hypocapnia with $Paco_2$ less than 38 mm Hg are associated with increased risk for CSBP.[17]

Patients may be asymptomatic, or may have complaints of daytime sleepiness, insomnia, nocturnal dyspnea, and/or other symptoms associated with the underlying medical disorder. CSBP is independently associated with an increased frequency of cardiac transplantation and risk of death in patients with CHF.[18]

Treatment

Continuous PAP
Summary of evidence There are several randomized controlled trials (RCTs) that address continuous PAP (CPAP) as a therapeutic modality for treatment of CSA in the setting of CSBP. However, CPAP was not titrated in many of these studies, making it difficult to determine response to treatment.

A post hoc analysis from the Canadian Positive Airway Pressure (CANPAP) trial, which consisted of 258 subjects with CHF and CSA, revealed that left ventricular ejection fraction (LVEF) and transplant-free survival rates were higher at the end of 3 months for the 57 subjects in whom

CSA was suppressed on CPAP (defined as AHI less than 15 per hour), compared with the controls and in the 43 patients in whom CSA was not suppressed on CPAP.[4,19] Another study of 66 patients with CHF showed a relative risk reduction of 81% (95% confidence interval [CI], 26%–95%) in combined mortality and cardiac transplantation rates at 2.2 years with CPAP use in the 29 patients with CSA/CSBP, but no effect in the 37 patients without CSA/CSBP.[20]

A meta-analysis of 7 studies, 6 of which were RCTs, showed that LVEF improved by a mean of 6% (95% CI, 2.4%–10.5%) in CPAP users versus controls. Another meta-analysis of 8 studies including 4 RCTs, 1 nonrandomized trial, and 3 others with data before and after commencing CPAP showed a mean reduction in AHI of 30 per hour (95% CI, 23–37), but with a mean residual AHI of 15 ± 4 per hour.[2]

Discussion Overall, when CSAS is adequately suppressed, CPAP seems to have a positive effect on transplant-free survival. Consistent effects on improvement in LVEF and AHI have been noted with CPAP in patients in whom CSAS is suppressed; however, not all patients respond to CPAP.

Recommendation "CPAP therapy targeted to normalize the AHI is indicated for the initial treatment of CSAS related to CHF."[2]

Level of recommendation Standard.[2]

Bilevel PAP

Summary of evidence In a small RCT comparing 10 cases on bilevel PAP (BPAP) in the spontaneous mode (BPAP-S) along with standard medical therapy with 11 controls on standard medical therapy alone, improvements in AHI, LVEF, and survival were reported over a mean of 31 ± 2.3 months.[21] However, BPAP-S can potentially precipitate or worsen central apneas and periodic breathing.

Two studies with 7 subjects each showed an improvement in LVEF by 12.7% $\pm$ 10% and 9.9% $\pm$ 9% respectively with BPAP in the spontaneous timed mode (BPAP-ST).[22,23] A meta-analysis of 3 studies evaluating before and after treatment effects of BPAP-ST showed a mean reduction in AHI of 44 per hour (95% CI, 40–49), with a residual AHI of less than 10 per hour.[2]

In a 14-day randomized crossover trial comparing BPAP-ST with CPAP in 16 patients with CHF, both devices were equally effective in improving New York Heart Association class and AHI.[24]

Discussion There is insufficient literature on the use of BPAP-S for CSA/CSBP. There is less research supporting the use of BPAP-ST compared with CPAP, adaptive servoventilation (ASV), or oxygen for these conditions, and BPAP-ST is typically more expensive than CPAP, calling into question the value of its use.

Recommendation "BPAP therapy in a spontaneous timed (ST) mode targeted to normalize the AHI may be considered for the treatment of CSAS related to CHF only if there is no response to adequate trials of CPAP, ASV, and oxygen therapies."[2]

Level of recommendation Option.[2]

ASV

Summary of evidence There are some studies, many of which are industry sponsored, comparing ASV treatment with baseline, subtherapeutic ASV, CPAP, BPAP-ST, and oxygen. A meta-analysis of 6 studies, including 4 RCTs with a total of 95 subjects assessing ASV effects on LVEF, showed an improvement by 6% (95% CI, 4%–8%).[2] In 2 of these studies ASV, but not CPAP, was seen to significantly increase LVEF over 3 to 6 months.[25,26] Another meta-analysis including 9 studies and 127 patients revealed a decrease in AHI with ASV by 31 (95% CI, 25–36) and 12 to 23 per hour compared with baseline and CPAP respectively. AHI was seen to normalize with ASV in most of the studies.[2] Subsequent studies have confirmed these effects on LVEF and AHI with ASV treatment.[27,28]

Two studies showed equivalent improvements in AHI with ASV and BPAP-ST[29,30] and 1 study showed that ASV was significantly better than oxygen at decreasing AHI in subjects with CSA.[31]

Discussion There are no long-term data on survival with ASV treatment of CSA/CSR. AHI and LVEF have shown consistent improvements with ASV, possibly greater than with CPAP, and there is even some evidence suggesting better compliance with ASV versus CPAP.[26] In contrast, ASV is more expensive and less easily available than CPAP. There is limited ability to generalize these research findings because of the different device algorithms in use and, in general, experience with the device is limited compared with CPAP.[2]

Recommendation "ASV targeted to normalize the AHI is indicated for the treatment of CSAS related to CSBP."[2]

Level of recommendation Standard.[2]

Oxygen

Summary of evidence Several studies have reported improvements in LVEF and AHI with oxygen therapy; however, the duration of follow-up is variable. A meta-analysis including 3 studies with a minimum follow-up period of 3 months, including 2 RCTs, showed a mean increase in LVEF of 5% (95% CI, 0.3%–9.8%) with oxygen treatment.[2]

Multiple studies have shown improvements in AHI in patients with CSA/CSBP with the use of oxygen. However, not all patients respond to oxygen.[32] A meta-analysis of 3 RCTs showed a mean reduction in AHI by 15 per hour (95% CI, 7–23) in 42 subjects using oxygen compared with 42 controls.[2]

In addition, improvement in other outcomes such as quality-of-life measures,[33] sleep architecture,[34] exercise capacity,[33,34] brain natriuretic peptide levels,[35] and sympathetic nerve activity[36] have been noted with oxygen treatment in some studies, with no reported long-term adverse effects.

Discussion There are no studies addressing mortality in patients with CSA/CSBP on oxygen therapy. One study showed no difference in cardiac events in subjects using oxygen versus those not on oxygen.[37] Evidence points toward improvement in LVEF and AHI with oxygen treatment, although to a lesser degree than with PAP. Oxygen treatment is expensive but is easily available, and hence may be considered in patients who find PAP therapy difficult to tolerate.

Recommendation "Nocturnal oxygen therapy is indicated for the treatment of CSAS related to CHF."[2]

Level of recommendation Standard.[2]

Treatment comparison studies

Summary of evidence In studies directly comparing the effectiveness of CPAP, BPAP, ASV, and oxygen treatments for CSAS, all modalities decrease AHI. However, BPAP seems to be better than CPAP. ASV seems to be equivalent to or possibly better than CPAP and BPAP-ST, particularly in patients with CSBP.[38–40]

Cardiac interventions

Summary of evidence Meta-analyses evaluating the effects of cardiac resynchronization therapy (CRT) in CSAS have shown improvement in LVEF by 8% (95% CI, 5%–12%) and AHI by 12 per hour (95% CI, 9–14).[2] No significant improvement has been shown with the addition of atrial overdrive pacing (AOP) compared with CRT.[41]

In one RCT that discussed the association between heart transplant and CSAS in 22 patients with CHF, CSAS persisted in some subjects despite normalization of cardiac function.[42]

Discussion Interventions including CRT, AOP, and cardiac transplantation can improve CSA by treating CHF. These procedures are expensive, require specialized skills, and have significant associated morbidity. Hence, treatment of CSA by itself is not considered an indication for these interventions.

Alternate therapies

Summary of evidence In one randomized crossover study, a statistically significant improvement in AHI but not LVEF was noted with acetazolamide.[43] Two studies that reported on the use of theophylline for CSA in the setting of CHF showed similar findings.[44,45]

Other studies have reported improvement in AHI with captopril and carvedilol, but the decrease in CSA may be secondary to improved cardiac function with the use of these agents.[46,47] There is scant evidence on the use of erythropoietin and intravenous iron in patients with CHF and anemia. Although carbon dioxide has been shown to possibly improve AHI in patients with CSA/CSBP in research settings,[48,49] the overall number of subjects was small. As noted previously, carbon dioxide is limited in availability and difficult to administer.

Discussion Overall, there is sparse evidence on the effects of alternate therapies in CSAS. Medications such as acetazolamide and theophylline have some evidence for use but are associated with significant adverse effects.

Recommendation "The following therapies have limited supporting evidence but may be considered for the treatment of CSAS related to CHF, after optimization of standard medical therapy, if PAP therapy is not tolerated, and if accompanied by close clinical follow-up: acetazolamide and theophylline."[2]

Level of recommendation Option.[2]

CSA DUE TO HIGH-ALTITUDE PERIODIC BREATHING
Definition

The ICSD-2 defines this disorder as recent ascent to altitude of at least 4000 m and polysomnography showing recurrent central apneas primarily during NREM sleep at a frequency of greater than 5 per hour. The cycle length should be between 12 and 34 seconds.[1]

Features

High-altitude periodic breathing (HAPB) is more likely to occur with rapid ascent to altitude and is seen in almost all individuals at altitudes of more than 7600 m. It is reported to be more common in men.[50]

Increased ventilatory chemoresponsiveness to hypoxia seems to be the main predisposing factor. Hyperventilation at high altitude induces respiratory alkalosis. The low Pa_{CO_2} results in a loss of respiratory drive during sleep when the apnea threshold is lowered. Breathing generally improves during REM sleep, possibly because of decreased hypoxic and hypercapnic chemoresponsiveness.[28,51]

Symptoms may include frequent awakenings, poor-quality sleep, feelings of breathlessness or suffocation, and fatigue or sleepiness. There is no clear association between this disorder and other altitude syndromes such as acute mountain sickness. Breathing becomes more regular with time at moderate altitude, but may persist indefinitely at high altitude.

Treatment

Summary of evidence

There are only 3 studies addressing the effects of pharmacologic agents on HAPB. Theophylline was equally effective as acetazolamide in normalizing AHI, but not for improving oxygen saturation.[52] Temazepam decreased time spent in periodic breathing but slightly decreased oxygen saturation.[53] No change in ventilatory parameters was noted with zolpidem and zaleplon versus placebo at simulated high altitude.[54]

Discussion

The low level of evidence precluded any recommendations for treatment in the practice parameters.[2]

CSA CAUSED BY MEDICAL CONDITIONS OTHER THAN CHEYNE-STOKES

This category includes patients with brainstem lesions that may be vascular, neoplastic, degenerative, demyelinating, or traumatic in origin, as well as cardiac and renal disorders that are not listed earlier.[1]

Treatment

Summary of evidence

There are 4 studies of treatment options for CSA in end-stage renal disease, all with significant limitations. Supplemental oxygen improved AHI and oxyhemoglobin saturation parameters in peritoneal dialysis patients with sleep disordered breathing (SDB) in 1 study.[55] Similar results were seen with CPAP for 1 night in subjects with renal failure and central/mixed apnea.[56] Fewer central apneas have been reported with bicarbonate buffer compared with acetate buffer[57] and with nocturnal dialysis compared with conventional hemodialysis.[58]

Discussion

The overall level of evidence for treatments of CSA in the setting of renal disease is currently low. Further research is needed to examine the relative risks and benefits of various modalities of treatment such as PAP and supplemental oxygen.

Recommendation

"The following possible treatment options for CSAS related to end-stage renal disease may be considered: CPAP, supplemental oxygen, bicarbonate buffer use during dialysis, and nocturnal dialysis."[2]

Level of recommendation Option.[2]

CSA CAUSED BY A DRUG OR SUBSTANCE

Definition

The ICSD-2 defines CSA caused by a drug or substance as a disorder that occurs in a patient taking a long-acting opioid regularly for at least 2 months, with polysomnography showing a central apnea index (CAI) of 5 or more, or periodic breathing (10 or more central apneas and hypopneas per hour of sleep in which the hyperpnea has a crescendo-decrescendo pattern of tidal volume, accompanied by frequent arousals from sleep and derangement of sleep structure), and the disorder is not better explained by another current sleep disorder or medical or neurologic disorder.[1]

Features

This disorder is most commonly reported with methadone, but is also seen with other opioids such as morphine, fentanyl, hydrocodone, and oxycodone.[59,60] Other respiratory disturbances such as obstructive hypoventilation, Biot breathing (**Fig. 2**), and cluster breathing (**Fig. 3**) may also occur.[61]

These drugs act on the mu receptors in the medulla causing depression of the hypercapnic ventilatory drive; this effect may improve after months of continued use.[62] Hypoxic ventilatory drive also seems to be increased.[63] The presence of abnormal breathing patterns during sleep in patients with chronic opioid use may suggest increased mortality.[64]

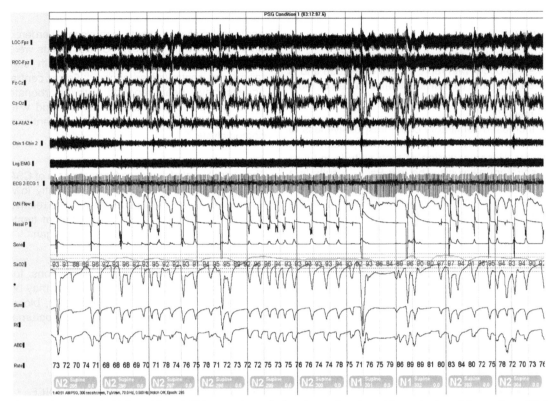

Fig. 2. Biot/nonperiodic breathing. A 300-second epoch showing a chaotic and irregular breathing pattern (Biot or ataxic breathing pattern) in a patient using chronic methadone for chronic pain syndrome.

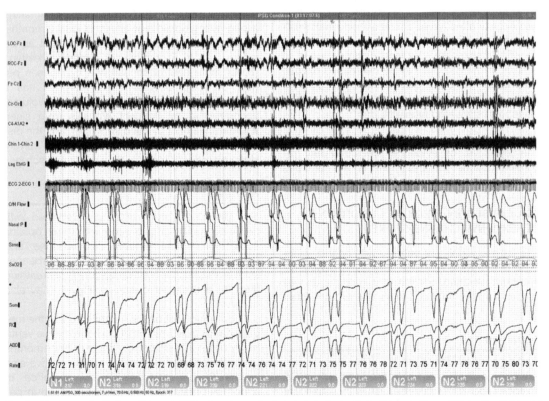

Fig. 3. Cluster periodic breathing. A 300-second epoch showing a cluster breathing pattern (2 breaths followed by an apnea) in a patient using methadone for chronic pain syndrome.

Treatment

Summary of evidence

There are limited data on treatment of CSAS caused by drugs or substances. In a study of 4 subjects with chronic pain on opioids who had CSA that was nonresponsive to CPAP, BPAP treatment of 6 months decreased the AHI and improved sleep fragmentation and hypoxemia.[65] A study by Allam and colleagues[39] in which 5 patients on opioids were included in the results suggested that ASV could be used as a therapeutic option. AHI was noted to decrease with CPAP as well as ASV in another study of 5 patients. CAI decreased to 0 on ASV and increased with CPAP but there was no effect on hypopneas.[66] In contrast, neither CPAP nor ASV changed AHI in a study of 22 subjects on chronic opioid treatment referred for suspected sleep apnea; the CAI did not decrease with ASV.[67] The difference in titration methods between the two studies may explain the differing results.

Discussion

The overall low level of evidence precluded treatment recommendations in the practice parameters.[2]

SUMMARY

Although current evidence suggests reasonable treatment of CSAS with PAP therapy, further long-term studies are required to address the effects on hospital admission rates, morbidity, and mortality. Also, additional studies comparing the relative cost-effectiveness, risks, and benefits of various treatment modalities are needed. More research on multimodality titration polysomnograms that use a different device when the previous one is unsuccessful may eventually help reduce testing time and health care costs.

Complex sleep apnea, the persistence or worsening of central sleep disordered breathing events on PAP in a patient with predominantly obstructive sleep apnea, was not addressed separately in the ICSD-2 or AASM practice parameters, but is a condition that is being increasingly encountered in clinical practice. Research is urgently desired to determine the need for and efficacy of treatment options for complex sleep apnea, particularly in the long term. At present, there is a paucity of literature on pharmacologic treatments for CSAS, especially CSAS not caused by CHF. Further studies are needed to evaluate the long-term harms and benefits of these treatments as well as new therapies such as exercise therapy and novel ventilation devices.

REFERENCES

1. The international classification of sleep disorders: diagnostic and coding manual. 2nd edition. Westchester (IL): American Academy of Sleep Medicine; 2005.
2. Aurora RN, Chowdhuri S, Ramar K, et al. The treatment of central sleep apnea syndromes in adults: practice parameters with an evidence-based literature review and meta-analyses. Sleep 2012;35: 17–40.
3. Guyatt GH, Oxman AD, Schunemann HJ, et al. GRADE guidelines: a new series of articles in the Journal of Clinical Epidemiology. J Clin Epidemiol 2011;64:380–2.
4. Bradley TD, McNicholas WT, Rutherford R, et al. Clinical and physiologic heterogeneity of the central sleep apnea syndrome. Am Rev Respir Dis 1986;134:217–21.
5. Xie A, Wong B, Phillipson EA, et al. Interaction of hyperventilation and arousal in the pathogenesis of idiopathic central sleep apnea. Am J Respir Crit Care Med 1994;150:489–95.
6. Xie A, Rutherford R, Rankin F, et al. Hypocapnia and increased ventilatory responsiveness in patients with idiopathic central sleep apnea. Am J Respir Crit Care Med 1995;152:1950–5.
7. Guilleminault C, Robinson A. Central sleep apnea. Neurol Clin 1996;14:611–28.
8. White DP, Zwillich CW, Pickett CK, et al. Central sleep apnea. Improvement with acetazolamide therapy. Arch Intern Med 1982;142:1816–9.
9. DeBacker WA, Verbraecken J, Willemen M, et al. Central apnea index decreases after prolonged treatment with acetazolamide. Am J Respir Crit Care Med 1995;151:87–91.
10. Quadri S, Drake C, Hudgel DW. Improvement of idiopathic central sleep apnea with zolpidem. J Clin Sleep Med 2009;5:122–9.
11. Bonnet MH, Dexter JR, Arand DL. The effect of triazolam on arousal and respiration in central sleep apnea patients. Sleep 1990;13:31–41.
12. Xie A, Rankin F, Rutherford R, et al. Effects of inhaled CO_2 and added dead space on idiopathic central sleep apnea. J Appl Physiol 1997;82:918–26.
13. Hall MJ, Xie A, Rutherford R, et al. Cycle length of periodic breathing in patients with and without heart failure. Am J Respir Crit Care Med 1996; 154:376–81.
14. Solin P, Roebuck T, Johns DP, et al. Peripheral and central ventilatory responses in central sleep apnea with and without congestive heart failure. Am J Respir Crit Care Med 2000;162:2194–200.
15. Xie A, Skatrud JB, Puleo DS, et al. Apnea-hypopnea threshold for CO_2 in patients with congestive heart failure. Am J Respir Crit Care Med 2002;165: 1245–50.

16. Naughton M, Benard D, Tam A, et al. Role of hyperventilation in the pathogenesis of central sleep apneas in patients with congestive heart failure. Am Rev Respir Dis 1993;148:330–8.

17. Sin DD, Fitzgerald F, Parker JD, et al. Risk factors for central and obstructive sleep apnea in 450 men and women with congestive heart failure. Am J Respir Crit Care Med 1999;160:1101–6.

18. Lanfranchi PA, Braghiroli A, Bosimini E, et al. Prognostic value of nocturnal Cheyne-Stokes respiration in chronic heart failure. Circulation 1999;99: 1435–40.

19. Arzt M, Floras JS, Logan AG, et al. Suppression of central sleep apnea by continuous positive airway pressure and transplant-free survival in heart failure: a post hoc analysis of the Canadian Continuous Positive Airway Pressure for Patients with Central Sleep Apnea and Heart Failure Trial (CANPAP). Circulation 2007;115:3173–80.

20. Sin DD, Logan AG, Fitzgerald FS, et al. Effects of continuous positive airway pressure on cardiovascular outcomes in heart failure patients with and without Cheyne-Stokes respiration. Circulation 2000;102:61–6.

21. Noda A, Izawa H, Asano H, et al. Beneficial effect of bilevel positive airway pressure on left ventricular function in ambulatory patients with idiopathic dilated cardiomyopathy and central sleep apnea-hypopnea: a preliminary study. Chest 2007;131: 1694–701.

22. Dohi T, Kasai T, Narui K, et al. Bi-level positive airway pressure ventilation for treating heart failure with central sleep apnea that is unresponsive to continuous positive airway pressure. Circ J 2008; 72:1100–5.

23. Kasai T, Narui K, Dohi T, et al. Efficacy of nasal bilevel positive airway pressure in congestive heart failure patients with Cheyne-Stokes respiration and central sleep apnea. Circ J 2005;69:913–21.

24. Kohnlein T, Welte T, Tan LB, et al. Assisted ventilation for heart failure patients with Cheyne-Stokes respiration. Eur Respir J 2002;20:934–41.

25. Philippe C, Stoica-Herman M, Drouot X, et al. Compliance with and effectiveness of adaptive servoventilation versus continuous positive airway pressure in the treatment of Cheyne-Stokes respiration in heart failure over a six month period. Heart 2006;92:337–42.

26. Kasai T, Usui Y, Yoshioka T, et al. Effect of flow-triggered adaptive servo-ventilation compared with continuous positive airway pressure in patients with chronic heart failure with coexisting obstructive sleep apnea and Cheyne-Stokes respiration. Circ Heart Fail 2010;3:140–8.

27. Koyama T, Watanabe H, Kobukai Y, et al. Beneficial effects of adaptive servo ventilation in patients with chronic heart failure. Circ J 2010;74:2118–24.

28. Goldberg SV, Schoene RB, Haynor D, et al. Brain tissue pH and ventilatory acclimatization to high altitude. J Appl Physiol 1992;72:58–63.

29. Fietze I, Blau A, Glos M, et al. Bi-level positive pressure ventilation and adaptive servo ventilation in patients with heart failure and Cheyne-Stokes respiration. Sleep Med 2008;9:652–9.

30. Morgenthaler TI, Gay PC, Gordon N, et al. Adaptive servoventilation versus noninvasive positive pressure ventilation for central, mixed, and complex sleep apnea syndromes. Sleep 2007;30:468–75.

31. Zhang XL, Yin KS, Jiang SS, et al. Efficacy of adaptive pressure support servo-ventilation in patients with congestive heart failure and Cheyne-Stokes respiration. Zhonghua Yi Xue Za Zhi 2006;86: 1620–3.

32. Javaheri S, Ahmed M, Parker TJ, et al. Effects of nasal O_2 on sleep-related disordered breathing in ambulatory patients with stable heart failure. Sleep 1999;22:1101–6.

33. Brostrom A, Hubbert L, Jakobsson P, et al. Effects of long-term nocturnal oxygen treatment in patients with severe heart failure. J Cardiovasc Nurs 2005; 20:385–96.

34. Staniforth AD, Kinnear WJ, Starling R, et al. Effect of oxygen on sleep quality, cognitive function and sympathetic activity in patients with chronic heart failure and Cheyne-Stokes respiration. Eur Heart J 1998;19:922–8.

35. Shigemitsu M, Nishio K, Kusuyama T, et al. Nocturnal oxygen therapy prevents progress of congestive heart failure with central sleep apnea. Int J Cardiol 2007;115:354–60.

36. Toyama T, Seki R, Kasama S, et al. Effectiveness of nocturnal home oxygen therapy to improve exercise capacity, cardiac function and cardiac sympathetic nerve activity in patients with chronic heart failure and central sleep apnea. Circ J 2009;73: 299–304.

37. Sasayama S, Izumi T, Matsuzaki M, et al. Improvement of quality of life with nocturnal oxygen therapy in heart failure patients with central sleep apnea. Circ J 2009;73:1255–62.

38. Hu K, Li QQ, Yang J, et al. The role of high-frequency jet ventilation in the treatment of Cheyne-Stokes respiration in patients with chronic heart failure. Int J Cardiol 2006;106:224–31.

39. Allam JS, Olson EJ, Gay PC, et al. Efficacy of adaptive servoventilation in treatment of complex and central sleep apnea syndromes. Chest 2007;132: 1839–46.

40. Teschler H, Dohring J, Wang YM, et al. Adaptive pressure support servo-ventilation: a novel treatment for Cheyne-Stokes respiration in heart failure. Am J Respir Crit Care Med 2001;164:614–9.

41. Luthje L, Renner B, Kessels R, et al. Cardiac resynchronization therapy and atrial overdrive

pacing for the treatment of central sleep apnoea. Eur J Heart Fail 2009;11:273–80.

42. Mansfield DR, Solin P, Roebuck T, et al. The effect of successful heart transplant treatment of heart failure on central sleep apnea. Chest 2003;124:1675–81.

43. Javaheri S. Acetazolamide improves central sleep apnea in heart failure: a double-blind, prospective study. Am J Respir Crit Care Med 2006;173:234–7.

44. Javaheri S, Parker TJ, Wexler L, et al. Effect of theophylline on sleep-disordered breathing in heart failure. N Engl J Med 1996;335:562–7.

45. Hu K, Li Q, Yang J, et al. The effect of theophylline on sleep-disordered breathing in patients with stable chronic congestive heart failure. Chin Med J (Engl) 2003;116:1711–6.

46. Tamura A, Kawano Y, Kadota J. Carvedilol reduces the severity of central sleep apnea in chronic heart failure. Circ J 2009;73:295–8.

47. Walsh JT, Andrews R, Starling R, et al. Effects of captopril and oxygen on sleep apnoea in patients with mild to moderate congestive cardiac failure. Br Heart J 1995;73:237–41.

48. Andreas S, Weidel K, Hagenah G, et al. Treatment of Cheyne-Stokes respiration with nasal oxygen and carbon dioxide. Eur Respir J 1998;12:414–9.

49. Steens RD, Millar TW, Su X, et al. Effect of inhaled 3% CO_2 on Cheyne-Stokes respiration in congestive heart failure. Sleep 1994;17:61–8.

50. Anholm JD, Powles AC, Downey R 3rd, et al. Operation Everest II: arterial oxygen saturation and sleep at extreme simulated altitude. Am Rev Respir Dis 1992;145:817–26.

51. Lahiri S, Maret K, Sherpa MG. Dependence of high altitude sleep apnea on ventilatory sensitivity to hypoxia. Respir Physiol 1983;52:281–301.

52. Fischer R, Lang SM, Leitl M, et al. Theophylline and acetazolamide reduce sleep-disordered breathing at high altitude. Eur Respir J 2004;23:47–52.

53. Nickol AH, Leverment J, Richards P, et al. Temazepam at high altitude reduces periodic breathing without impairing next-day performance: a randomized cross-over double-blind study. J Sleep Res 2006;15:445–54.

54. Beaumont M, Batejat D, Coste O, et al. Effects of zolpidem and zaleplon on sleep, respiratory patterns and performance at a simulated altitude of 4,000 m. Neuropsychobiology 2004;49:154–62.

55. Kumagai T, Ishibashi Y, Kawarazaki H, et al. Effects of nocturnal oxygen therapy on sleep apnea syndrome in peritoneal dialysis patients. Clin Nephrol 2008;70:332–9.

56. Pressman MR, Benz RL, Schleifer CR, et al. Sleep disordered breathing in ESRD: acute beneficial effects of treatment with nasal continuous positive airway pressure. Kidney Int 1993;43:1134–9.

57. Jean G, Piperno D, Francois B, et al. Sleep apnea incidence in maintenance hemodialysis patients: influence of dialysate buffer. Nephron 1995;71:138–42.

58. Hanly PJ, Pierratos A. Improvement of sleep apnea in patients with chronic renal failure who undergo nocturnal hemodialysis. N Engl J Med 2001;344:102–7.

59. Teichtahl H, Prodromidis A, Miller B, et al. Sleep-disordered breathing in stable methadone programme patients: a pilot study. Addiction 2001;96:395–403.

60. Walker JM, Farney RJ, Rhondeau SM, et al. Chronic opioid use is a risk factor for the development of central sleep apnea and ataxic breathing. J Clin Sleep Med 2007;3:455–61.

61. Farney RJ, Walker JM, Cloward TV, et al. Sleep-disordered breathing associated with long-term opioid therapy. Chest 2003;123:632–9.

62. Shook JE, Watkins WD, Camporesi EM. Differential roles of opioid receptors in respiration, respiratory disease, and opiate-induced respiratory depression. Am Rev Respir Dis 1990;142:895–909.

63. Teichtahl H, Wang D, Cunnington D, et al. Ventilatory responses to hypoxia and hypercapnia in stable methadone maintenance treatment patients. Chest 2005;128:1339–47.

64. Webster LR, Cochella S, Dasgupta N, et al. An analysis of the root causes for opioid-related overdose deaths in the United States. Pain Med 2011;12(Suppl 2):S26–35.

65. Alattar MA, Scharf SM. Opioid-associated central sleep apnea: a case series. Sleep Breath 2009;13:201–6.

66. Javaheri S, Malik A, Smith J, et al. Adaptive pressure support servoventilation: a novel treatment for sleep apnea associated with use of opioids. J Clin Sleep Med 2008;4:305–10.

67. Farney RJ, Walker JM, Boyle KM, et al. Adaptive servoventilation (ASV) in patients with sleep disordered breathing associated with chronic opioid medications for non-malignant pain. J Clin Sleep Med 2008;4:311–9.

Cheyne-Stokes Respiration

Matthew T. Naughton, MBBS, MD, FRACP

KEYWORDS

- Cheyne-Stokes respiration • Central sleep apnea • Heart failure

KEY POINTS

- Cheyne-Stokes respiration (CSR) is a disorder of hyperventilation usually in the setting of moderate to severe congestive heart failure. The cycle length (of apnea and hyperpnea) is characteristically greater than 45 seconds in duration and can be used to distinguish CSR caused by cardiac disease from other forms of central sleep apnea such as that seen with narcotics for which the cycle length is less than 45 seconds.
- Measures of hypoxemia, heart rate, and loop gain (eg, ratio of ventilation length/apnea length) during sleep may more reliably indicate CSR severity than simply the apnea-hypopnea index. The apnea-hypopnea index was designed to measure severity of obstructive sleep apnea, not CSR.
- The most effective forms of treatment of CSR are those directed at the cause, namely the heart condition (either the pump, the valves, or the rhythm and rate). This treatment may involve medications, valve replacement, or other mechanical treatments such as pacemakers. One treatment strategy sleep services have to offer is continuous positive airway pressure (CPAP), which helps some types of heart failure. Whether newer forms of CPAP, such as adaptive servo-controlled ventilation, which attempts to provide ventilatory support during the apneas while reducing overall minute ventilation and allowing CO_2 levels to increase, has any long-term additional benefit remains to be proved.

INTRODUCTION

Central sleep apnea (CSA) is a broad descriptive term for apneas during sleep that result from altered respiratory drive. Two categories exist[1]: the first is defined by abnormal nocturnal hypoventilation and hypercapnia ($Paco_2$ evening to morning change >5 mm Hg), which can result from various musculoskeletal, neuromuscular, or neurologic disorders such as kyphoscoliosis, syringomyelia, myotonic dystrophy, or obesity hypoventilation syndrome. This category is not discussed any further in this article.

The second category relates to transient, cyclic, or periodic loss of respiratory drive, interspersed with brief periods of hyperventilation, usually associated with normocapnia or hypocapnia ($Paco_2$<45 mm Hg). This second type of CSA can be caused by conditions such as heart failure (HF) (in which it is known as Cheyne-Stokes

respiration [CSR]), narcotic drugs, continuous positive airway pressure (CPAP; also known as complex CSA), premature infancy, and high altitude. This article focuses on the CSA with CSR (CSA-CSR) seen in HF.

EPIDEMIOLOGY

Approximately 70% of the population with HF has a sleep-related breathing disorder (SRBD), as defined by an apnea-hypopnea index (AHI) of more than 5 events per hour.[2–4] This generalized SRBD persists when clinic patients with routine HF have repeated cardiopulmonary studies over a 12-month period.[5] The SRBD group can be further categorized into 2 groups: one with predominantly obstructive sleep apnea (OSA), the second with predominantly CSA-CSR. OSA is considered a cause of HF, whereas CSA-CSR is considered a result of HF.[6]

Department of Allergy, Immunology and Respiratory Medicine, Alfred Hospital, Monash University, Melbourne, 55 Commercial Road, Victoria 3004, Australia
E-mail address: m.naughton@alfred.org.au

Sleep Med Clin 9 (2014) 13–25
http://dx.doi.org/10.1016/j.jsmc.2013.11.002
1556-407X/14/$ – see front matter © 2014 Elsevier Inc. All rights reserved.

HF is a complex disorder caused by a broad range of conditions, an understanding of which is required to understand the pathogenesis and management of CSA-CSR. The diagnostic accuracy of tools commonly used to identify HF needs to be understood. For example, two-dimensional echocardiography is operator dependent and of limited averaging time, and has high variability compared with other markers of left ventricular function such as nuclear medicine techniques, which are three-dimensional and gated over several minutes. The clinician needs to understand the cause(s), duration, age of onset, and stability of HF in order to understand the symptoms and determine management of CSA-CSR. HF is commonly associated with hyponatremia, anemia, renal impairment, skeletal muscle wasting, malnutrition, neurohumoral changes, and psychiatric changes, the symptoms of which can overlap with SRBD symptoms. In addition, some features of HF, such as renal impairment, may interfere with the control of breathing, or anemia may aggravate periodic limb movements (PLMs) and dyspnea. Although stroke is a commonly proposed cause of CSA-CSR, the only study in which patients with stroke with CSA were assessed for cardiac dysfunction identified that hypocapnia and occult cardiac failure were strongly associated with CSA, rather than location or type of stroke.[7]

Although medical therapies directed toward HF severity, which should alleviate CSA-CSR, have advanced in the past 3 decades, the introduction of β-blockers and spironolactone has not altered the prevalence of CSA-CSR.[8,9]

PATHOPHYSIOLOGY

During wakefulness, ventilation is under cortical and metabolic control (ie, CO_2 sensed by the peripheral and central chemoreceptors).[9] During rapid eye movement (REM) sleep, ventilation is under pontomedullary inspiratory neuron control (ie, not metabolic), which is responsible for the characteristic irregular respiratory rate and tidal volume appearance. Ventilation during slow wave sleep is under metabolic control with increased CO_2 and arousal thresholds, which results in the characteristic stable ventilation pattern.

During the transition from wakefulness to stages 1 and 2 non-REM sleep, cortical control is diminished and ventilation becomes dependent on $Paco_2$ (**Fig. 1**).[10] In order to achieve this, minute ventilation transiently decreases (~20%) and accordingly the prevailing $Paco_2$ level increases (~2–3 mm Hg). A new $Paco_2$ and V steady state are reached and a regular respiratory pattern results in this new equilibrium during stable non-REM sleep. During non-REM stages N1 and N2, an unstable respiratory state can be precipitated by an arousal or change in sleep state (of any cause) resulting in the development of CSA-CSR. Ventilation transiently increases with arousal and is followed by a decrease in $Paco_2$, to a level less than the threshold required to stimulate ventilation. This change in $Paco_2$ is called the CO_2 reserve. A central apnea ensues (~30 seconds in HF), during which the $Paco_2$ level increases. A period of hyperventilation follows (~30 seconds), which drives the $Paco_2$ level to less than the threshold again, thereby precipitating a further central apnea. This cycle of hyperventilation followed by central apnea is called CSR. When hyperventilation is followed by cyclic hypopneas, the term periodic breathing is often used, and this pattern can be observed awake and often at the onset of exercise (when undergoing cardiopulmonary exercise testing).

CO₂ Reserve

Patients with CSA-CSR have a low prevailing CO_2 value[11,12] with an increased minute ventilation compared with HF without CSA-CSR. For example, in one study, the $Paco_2$ values were ~33 and ~38 mm Hg and minute volume of ventilation were ~8.3 versus 6.8 L/min in a CSA-CSR group compared with an HF group with normal ventilation.[11] The $Paco_2$ value may decrease by a further 1 to 2 mm Hg during the night, especially if the patient has both OSA and CSA-CSR.[13]

The transient oscillations in $Paco_2$ required to precipitate a central apnea is called the CO_2 reserve. The CO_2 reserve can be measured under experimental and artificial conditions by altering CO_2 with either noninvasive ventilation or addition of CO_2. Patients with HF without CSA-CSR have a CO_2 reserve of ~5 mm Hg for apnea development and ~4 mm Hg for hypopnea development.[14] In comparison, patients with HF with CSA-CSR, have CO_2 reserves of ~3 mm Hg and ~1.5 mm Hg for apnea and hypopnea development respectively.[14] Thus a large CO_2 reserve protects against CSA, whereas a small reserve may predispose to CSA-CSR.

It has been proposed that the CO_2 reserve can be manipulated. For example, metabolic acidosis, almitrine,[15] and clonidine[16] have been shown to increase the CO_2 reserve, whereas metabolic alkalosis and hypoxia have been shown to reduce the CO_2 reserve.[15] Whether this manipulation of CO_2 threshold has a therapeutic role remains to be determined.

Loop Gain

Loop gain is an engineering term that describes the cyclic behavior of an insult (eg, hyperventilation)

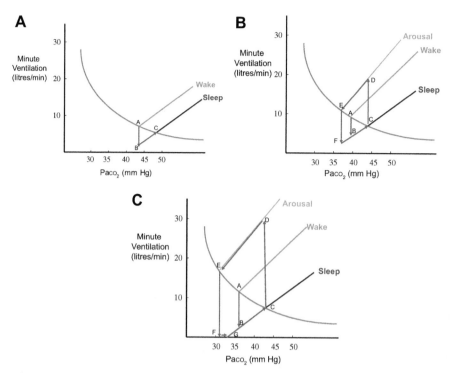

Fig. 1. The relationship between metabolic hyperbole and ventilatory responses during wakefulness, non-REM sleep, and arousal in (A) HF with normal ventilation, (B) HF with hypopneas, and (C) HF with CSA-CSR. Note that in normal ventilation (A), ventilation and $Paco_2$ when awake are situated at A and, with sleep onset, ventilation decreases and CO_2 increases (B) to reach a new equilibrium at C. In (B), note the introduction of arousal and the leftward shift of the wake and sleep ventilatory responses. With sleep onset, ventilation decreases and CO_2 level increases (A to B), and rests at C until an arousal occurs, transiently increasing ventilation to D, driving CO_2 down (D to E), which results in hypopnea (E to F) and resumption to C until a further arousal (C to D). In (C), ventilation decreases and CO_2 level increases with sleep onset (A to B), and resets at C until an arousal occurs, increasing ventilation to D, driving CO_2 down (D to E), which results in an apnea (F to G), then an increase in CO_2 to C. A further arousal increases ventilation (C to D) and so forth. (*From* Phillipson EA, Bradley TD. Central sleep apnea. Clin Chest Med 1992;13(3):493–505; with permission.)

followed by a disturbance (eg, central apnea). Several descriptions of loop gain exist, but this article focuses on 3 descriptions.

The first is the ratio of the ventilation length (VL) or duration divided by the following apnea length (AL) duration (VL/AL) taken directly from a polysomnogram. This ratio is useful to distinguish the CSA of a cardiac cause (VL/AL >1) from a noncardiac cause (VL/AL<1) (**Fig. 2**).[17] The VL/AL ratio can be complemented by the overall cycle length (CL = VL + AL), which is characteristically long in CSA of cardiac cause (45–90 seconds) compared with noncardiac causes (<45 seconds).[17,18]

The second description requires an estimate of duty ratio (DR), which is the VL/CL ratio, in which CL is cycle length, from which loop gain can be estimated as $2\pi/2\pi DR\text{-sin}(2\pi DR)$.[19] This method of loop gain is thought to predict responsiveness to treatments such as CPAP for CSA-CSR. For example, if loop gain is high, as estimated by DR

less than 0.7 and LG greater than 1.2, the CPAP responsiveness in terms of AHI reduction will be modest (0%–50 % reduction), whereas if DR is greater than 0.7 and LG less than 1.2, the AHI response to CPAP should be 50% to 100% effective.

The third loop gain concept has also been used to understand the interplay between the driver of the insult (controller; ie, the brain), the disturbance (plant; ie, the lungs), and the delay (feedback; ie, cardiac output).[20] In such terms, changes in either the controller, plant, or cardiac output can result in greater understanding of the mechanisms responsible for developing CSA-CSR. For example, if the controller has an increased output for a given signal (for example, an increased ventilatory response to CO_2),[21] controller gain has occurred and CSA-CSR may result. Alternatively, the disturbance may be exaggerated (ie, plant gain) by conditions such as pulmonary edema, cardiomegaly,

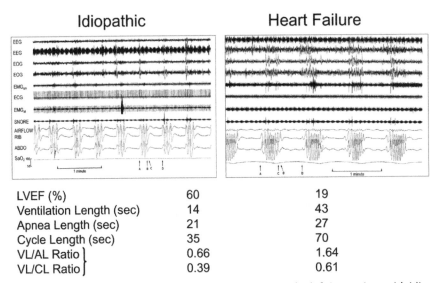

	Idiopathic	Heart Failure
LVEF (%)	60	19
Ventilation Length (sec)	14	43
Apnea Length (sec)	21	27
Cycle Length (sec)	35	70
VL/AL Ratio	0.66	1.64
VL/CL Ratio	0.39	0.61

Fig. 2. Two polysomnograms (4-minute page) of patients with CSA. On the left is a patient with idiopathic CSA in whom left ventricular ejection fraction (LVEF) is 60%. Note the short cycle length (~35 seconds), whereas the polysomnogram on the right represents a patient with typical CSA-CSR with a long cycle length (~70 seconds). Also note the differences in ventilation and apnea lengths and the ratios VL/AL and VL/CL.

and pleural effusions, which result in restrictive ventilatory defect and greater hypoxemia for a given apnea. Changes in lung function (discussed later) are more common in patients with CSA-CSR than in those without.[22]

Vagal Afferent

Instrumented feline studies suggested that, if the pulmonary artery pressure was artificially increased, ventilation rate would increase; an effect blocked by vagotomy.[23] Therefore it was concluded that conditions that can increase pulmonary artery pressure, such as HF, can trigger hyperventilation via pulmonary J receptors and vagal afferent nerves. Support for this is provided by the relationship between pulmonary capillary wedge pressure (PCWP) and AHI[4] and inversely with $Paco_2$.[24] Following HF treatment, PCWP decreases in parallel with an increase in $Paco_2$ and a decrease in AHI.[4,25] In addition, circumstantial evidence is provided by Yumino and colleagues[26] suggesting that the change in leg fluid volume (an index of rostral fluid shift) is proportional to the change in transcutaneous partial pressure of CO_2 ($PtcCO_2$) during sleep and increase in central AHI.

Although this mechanism may be operational, patients who are vagally denervated because of bilateral lung transplantation, and confirmed by heart rate variability studies, can still have CSA-CSR with the development of HF. Moreover, the control of HF paralleled the severity of CSA.[27] Thus mechanisms other than vagal afferents are operational.

Chemosensitivity

An increased chemosensitivity underpins CSA-CSR and results in hyperventilation awake, asleep, and even during exercise. Central and peripheral reflexes to CO_2 were increased in patients with HF with CSA-CSR in contrast with HF with OSA and normal ventilation.[21] Others have reported that PCWP correlates with $Paco_2$.[24] Mechanisms responsible for the increased chemosensitivity are understood to be increased sympathetic activity (related to degree of HF), increased vagal afferent activity, and loss of endothelial cells in the carotid body, which release nitric oxide.[28] There is increased sympathetic activity, as measured in urine,[29,30] plasma,[29] direct skeletal muscle sympathetic activity, and tritiated norepinephrine spillover,[31] which are increased in CSA-CSR compared with OSA and HF control subjects with normal ventilation.

Upper Airway

During CSA-CSR, the airway is either open throughout the apnea or open for the first half, closing midway **(Fig. 3)**.[32,33] The $PetCO_2$ measured during sleep can give an indirect signal as to the upper airway patency, with increased $PetCO_2$ during an apnea indicating an open airway (ie, a prolonged expiration), whereas $PetCO_2$ that is increased then decreases to zero midway through an apnea indicates closure of the airway. In ~50% of CSA-CSR apneas, the airway remains open, whereas in the remainder the airway closes during the apnea. If respiratory effort is carefully

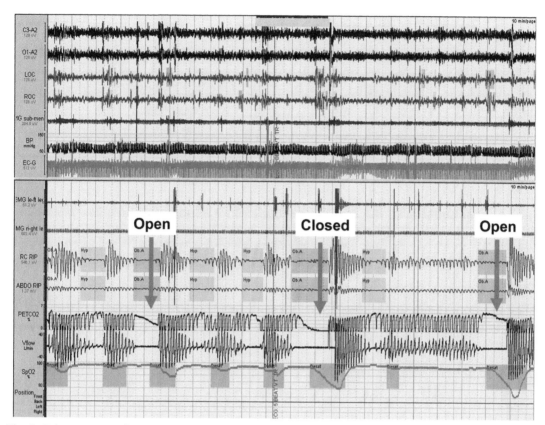

Fig. 3. Polysomnogram (10-minute page) of patient with CSA-CSR showing end-tidal P_{CO_2} with 2 open and 1 closed apneas.

assessed by esophageal manometry when the airway closes in CSA, 2 to 3 respiratory efforts are seen before airway opening, indicating a misalignment of respiratory effort and ventilation. The upper airway during CSA-CSR has not been well studied, although it seems that closure is passive[32,33] and may be influenced by rostral fluid shift contributing to upper airway edema. In contrast, diuresis may be effective in alleviating some of this upper airway closure. Although snoring is uncommon in CSA-CSR, it sometimes occurs during the peak of the hyperventilation period. CPAP may be useful in CSA-CSR to maintain upper airway patency and avoid futile respiratory effort at the end of apnea.

In addition, route of ventilation changes in normal subjects when exercising, and minute volume of ventilation (MVV) increases to more than 20 L/min.[34,35] At less than 20 L/min, nasal ventilation is usually adequate; whereas normal subjects initiate oral ventilation when MVV is greater than 20 L/min. The same is seen in CSA-CSR (**Fig. 4**) with oral breathing at peak ventilation. There are 2 clinical implications: the first is that hypopneas with some effort (ie, central hypopneas) can be

misclassified as obstructive apneas if nasal flow alone is measured without oral ventilation (see **Fig. 4**). Second, if tidal volumes are large and the patient needs to mouth breath, the choice of mask for positive airway pressure (oronasal vs nasal) is important. Patients with CSA-CSR often prefer oronasal masks when using positive airway pressure.

Change in CSA-CSR Overnight

The type of SRBD may change during the evening. Work by a group in Toronto indicated that patients with HF with both OSA and CSA-CSR may convert from an OSA-dominant pattern at the onset of sleep to a CSA-CSR-dominant pattern toward the end of the night.[13] The AHI caused by OSA decreased from ~69% to 23% of all events and CSA increased from ~31% to 78% without a change in overall AHI or position. Associated with this change in apnea type was an increase in MVV (~8 to 9.5 L/min), a decrease in $PtcCO_2$ (~42 to 39 mm Hg), and a lengthening of the lung-to-ear circulation time (21 to 24 seconds) and cycle length (~50 to 54 seconds).[13] These

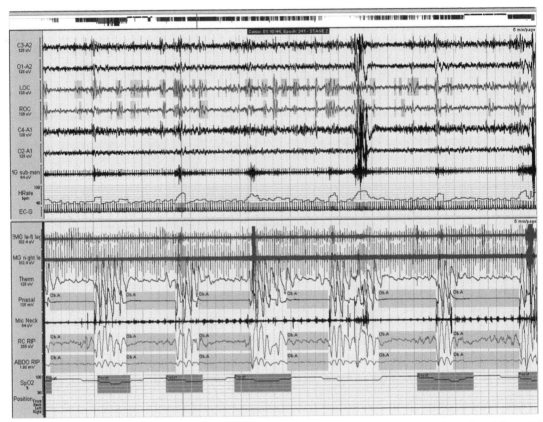

Fig. 4. Polysomnogram (5-minute page) showing absence of nasal pressure, but preservation of oral flow: this shows the difficulty in distinguishing central hypopnea from obstructive apnea.

findings strongly support the concept of a detrimental effect of OSA on cardiac function.

Additional support for this observation that OSA has a detrimental effect has recently been provided by the observation that obstructive apneas impair stroke volume, in contrast with central apneas, which do not reduce (and may improve) stroke volume.[36] This finding confirms animal work that showed that OSA causes reduced left ventricular function.[37] In contrast with the negative effects of OSA, CSA may not have the same adverse effects; there may be an increase in stroke volume with central apneas and hyperventilation.[36,38]

Our group has assessed heart rate and heart rate variability in patients with pure CSA-CSR and found that time of evening did not have an influence on any marker of cardiac autonomic control,[39] thereby suggesting that the presence of CSA-CSR, in contrast with OSA, does not result in an escalation of cardiac impairment through the night.

Pulmonary changes with HF

Pulmonary changes are also common in HF and need to be considered when dealing with the dyspneic patient.[40] Radiological evidence of cardiomegaly, interstitial edema, alveolar edema, and pleural effusions are common and assist in understanding the pulmonary physiologic tests that indicate restrictive ventilation defects with impaired diffusing capacity. Respiratory muscles are often weak, associated with global skeletal myopathy. Amiodarone and smoking may further impair lung function.

High-powered electron microscopy of the lung suggests interstitial edema, increased interstitial tissue hemosiderin deposition, alveolar wall thickening, and fibrosis of the pulmonary arteries, a remodeling process that is considered to be a protective mechanism against interstitial edema and alveolar edema, at the expense of right HF.[40]

During sleep, end-expiratory lung volume increases during the hyperventilation period[41,42] to a level of approximately 500 mL, which is equivalent to that seen with CPAP.

Cardiopulmonary exercise tests indicate a reduced peak workload, heightened ventilation to CO_2 production slope, a peak heart rate greater than 85% of predicted, ventilation less than 85%, and an absence of hypoxemia.

Body position (vertical and rotation)

It has been known for decades that HF often presents with orthopnea and paroxysmal nocturnal dyspnea. Studies of patients with HF with esophageal manometry during sleep conducted more than 60 years ago showed that elevating the head of the bed had a profound beneficial effect on CSA-CSR severity.[43] This effect of vertical change in body position on CSA-CSR is most likely related to increased lung volume and improved ventilation perfusion matching when upright compared with in a supine position.

More recently, lateral rotational movement has also been found to have a profound effect on CSA-CSR.[44–46] In one study,[46] the AHI decreased by ~50% when the patients' sleeping position was changed from supine to lateral. This change in position was associated with a diminished oxygen desaturation for a given AL (ie, less hypoxemia). Leung and colleagues[45] reported oxygen saturation via pulse oximetry (Spo$_2$) values to be similar in the left and right lateral positions, so there seems to be no identified difference in right compared with left positions. The investigators speculated that the postural effect of change in AHI and oxygenation are not related to the upper airway, but instead to changes in lung volume[47] or venous return.[48]

CLINICAL FEATURES OF CSA-CSR

Common symptoms of HF include dyspnea, cough, and fatigue, which overlap with CSA-CSR (**Box 1**). There is a wide spectrum of dyspnea severity from mild exertional dyspnea with strenuous activity, to extreme dyspnea with mild exertion, and dyspnea at rest, and orthopnea. Cough may be intermittent and dry, usually related to subacute pulmonary interstitial edema or possibly triggered by medications (classically angiotensin-converting enzyme inhibitors). Intermittent pink frothy sputum sometimes occurs because of alveolar edema. Fatigue may be associated with insomnia and lethargy rather than sleepiness,[49] probably related to degree of sympathetic activity offsetting sleepiness.

PLMs are common in HF and CSA-CSR. The PLMs have different cycle lengths to that of the respiration. Hanly and colleagues[50] assessed the impact of PLMs in a population with HF and observed that ~50% of patients with HF had a Periodic limb movement index (PLMI) greater than 25 events per hour, and PLMI was related to a reduced mean sleep latency test. Low iron levels and anemia, common in HF, may contribute to the development of restless legs. The response of CSA-CSR to treatment depends on whether the treatment is directed toward the cause (HF)

Box 1
Characteristic features of CSA-CSR

Advanced HF

  Reduced LVEF (if systolic HF)

  Increased pulmonary capillary wedge pressure

  Atrial fibrillation and tachyarrhythmias

  Large dilated left ventricle chamber

  Increased biomarkers (brain natriuretic peptide, atrial natriuretic peptide)

Polysomnogram

  Crescendo-decrescendo ventilatory pattern

  Apneas and hypopneas in stages N1 + N2 (and wake)

  Hyperventilation and hypocapnia

  Cycle length 45 to 75 seconds

Neurohumoral abnormalities

  Sympathetic activity increased

  Vagal activity decreased

  Increased brain natriuretic peptide

  Loss of nitric oxide

Clinical

  Men (>90%)

  Minimal snoring

  Orthopnea

  Fatigue

  Responsive to HF treatment

  Witnessed silent apneas

Pulmonary function

  Low Paco$_2$

  Restrictive ventilatory defect

  Reduced diffusing capacity

  Increased ventilatory response to CO_2

  Reduced maximal inspiratory and expiratory pressures (MIPS and MEPS)

  Reduced maximal oxygen consumption ($\dot{V}o_2$ max) with increased expired air flow ($\dot{V}_E$)/carbon dioxide production ($\dot{V}co_2$) and absence of hypoxemia

---

or to abolishing the AHI to fewer than 5 events per hour (**Table 1**). Note that the more effective and successful the treatment directed toward the underlying HF, the greater the improvement in AHI. In contrast, treatments directed specifically at the CSA-CSR alone (eg, dead space and inhaled CO_2) run the potential risk of abolishing the AHI to

Table 1
Comparison of treatments for HF and for CSA-CSR as defined by the AHI

Treatment	HF	CSA-CSR
HF medications		
BB, ACEI	++	++
Pacemakers		
Cardiac	+++	+++
Biventricular	+++	+++
Cardiac valve replacement	+++	+++
Left ventricular devices	+++	+++
Heart transplant	+++	+++
CPAP		
Fixed	+++	++
Adaptive	+++	++
Oxygen	-	+
Respiratory stimulants		
Acetazolamide	+	++
Theophylline	-	++
Inhaled CO_2	-	+++
Dead space	-	+++
Anxiolytics		
Benzodiazepines	-	+

-, no change; +, partial improvement possible; ++, major improvement possible; +++, major improvement likely.
   Abbreviations: ACEI, angiotensin-converting enzyme inhibitors; BB, β-blockers.

fewer than 5 events per hour with little, or possibly detrimental, impact on cardiac function.

MONITORING TECHNIQUES

CSA-CSR is characterized by a cyclic crescendo-decrescendo respiratory effort usually in the awake: stages N1 and N2 transition associated with an arousal at peak ventilation (**Fig. 5**). It is often precipitated by a large arousal, movement, or state change. The apnea-hyperpnea cycle length, 45 to 75 seconds, can assist in distinguishing CSA of HF cause from other causes (such as narcotic or CPAP induced).[17,51] CSA-CSR is usually worse in the supine position and can be alleviated by elevation of the head of the bed, or moving from supine to lateral body positions. Hypoxemia is variable, sometimes absent, or cyclic between 90% and 100% SpO_2. Although rarely measured in routine polysomnography, the overall minute ventilation is increased in CSA-CSR, as indicated by a prevailing hypocapnia and alkalosis. Systemic blood pressure and heart rate variability typically become entrained to the respiratory pattern (see **Fig. 5**). Sleep architecture is usually severely fragmented, with deficient stage N3 and REM sleep. PLMs commonly coexist, often with a different frequency to that of the CSA-CSR.

The distinction between subtypes of sleep disordered breathing (obstructive and CSA-CSR) critically depends on the techniques used during monitoring. However, variations in techniques and definitions used to describe sleep disordered breathing and the thresholds used to divide SRBD between mainly central and mainly obstructive have led to marked variations in reports.

Detailed monitoring (see **Figs. 2–5**) indicates that overlap between the two distinct entities (OSA and CSA-CSR) is commonplace. Moreover, the choice of monitoring must be made in conjunction with a detailed clinical examination and history (including bed partner) because this is frequently revealing in terms of snoring.

Ambulatory limited channel (eg, oximetry) and in-laboratory polysomnography have been used in published studies of CSA-CSR. Simple overnight oximetry, with ~2-second averaging times and less than 0.1-Hz sampling frequency, has a characteristic appearance (see **Fig. 5**A) with SpO_2 oscillating between 100% and 90%, without clear-cut periods of REM-related desaturation. One study[52] estimated a sensitivity and specificity of identifying SRBD (AHI>15 and oxygen desaturation index >10) to be 85% and 93% respectively against a gold standard of in-laboratory polysomnography performed on another night, but there was poor discrimination between OSA and CSA-CSR. Limitations to this technique are lack of body position, electrocardiogram rhythm, and respiratory effort in addition to other standard features with polysomnography. Other level 3 devices have been used, and may have improved differentiation of OSA from CSA-CSR.[53]

Laboratory-based polysomnography is useful for patients with HF because they may be unstable and need supervision. In addition, accurate estimations of body position (vertical and rotational), route of ventilation (oral vs nasal), cardiac rhythm and blood pressure, CO_2 (transcutaneous or arterial), respiratory effort (esophageal manometry), sleep architecture, and PLMs are essential to optimize management of patients with HF with possible sleep-related breathing disturbances.

By consensus[54] CSA-CSR is scored if both of the following are met: (1) there are episodes of at least 3 consecutive central apneas and/or central hypopneas separated by a crescendo and decrescendo change in breathing amplitude with a cycle length of at least 40 seconds (typically 45–90 seconds), and (2) there are 5 or more central apneas and/or central hypopneas per hour associated with the crescendo-decrescendo breathing

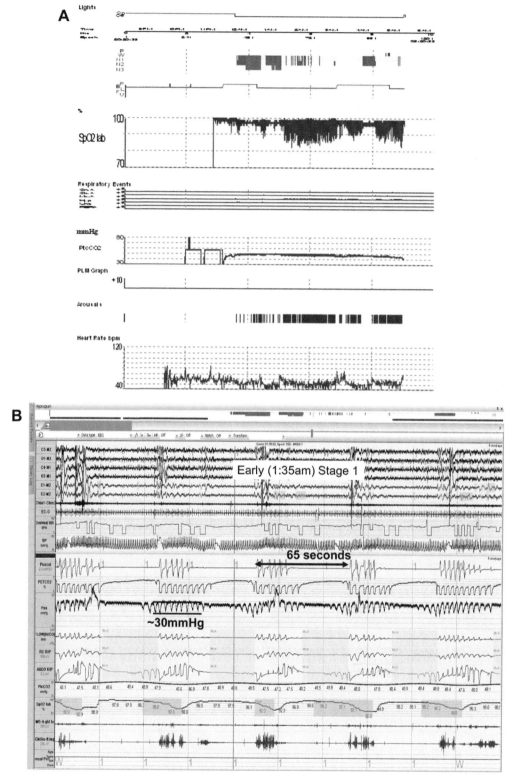

Fig. 5. Overnight polysomography with esophageal manometry, continuous systemic blood pressure, transcutaneous CO_2, end-tidal CO_2, and tidal volume in 54-year-old man with ischemic cardiomyopathy (LVEF, 20%). Body mass index was 36 kg/m², AHI was 40/h, minimum Spo_2 was 82%. (*A*) Overnight summary. (*B–D*) Five-minute pages. Evening and morning $Paco_2$ were 43 and 42 mm Hg respectively. Note the typical oximetry pattern on summary sheet (*A*) showing the oscillation in Spo_2 between 100% and 82%. Note that the 5-minute polysomnography shows typical CSA-CSR at the beginning (*B*) and end of the evening (*C*), showing no change in any physiologic parameter, including cycle length. Note that pleural pressure swings are less and periodic in CSA-CSR (*B, C*) compared with stable ventilation in stages N2 and N3 (*D*) sleep.

C

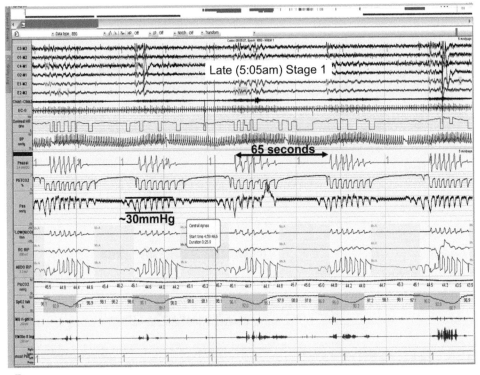

D

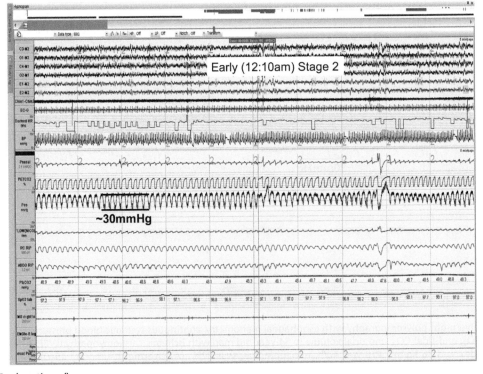

Fig. 5. (*continued*)

pattern recorded over a minimum of 2 hours of monitoring.

Is CSA-CSR Detrimental?

CSA-CSR is seen in severe HF.[55] This level of HF may or may not be reversible. Evidence in support of this is the relationship between CSA-CSR severity and markers of HF severity (eg, PCWP, brain natriuretic peptide, catecholamines). Whether CSA-CSR is associated with increased mortality, as suggested by some studies, or is causative, as suggested by other investigators, is a moot point.

The adverse effects of CSA-CSR are well described: fragmented sleep, intermittent hypoxia, increased sympathetic activity, hypocapnic cerebral vasoconstriction, and the associated features of atrial fibrillation and cardiac arrhythmias. However, these are associations rather than necessarily causative of increased mortality. Many patients with CSA-CSR are not hypoxemic.

An alternative view is that CSA-CSR brings benefits to a system exposed to recurring pulmonary edema: cyclic breathing provides periodic rest, and the hyperventilation phase is associated with an increase in end-expiratory lung volume.[41,42] Stroke volume is thought to be augmented by the periodicity of breathing.[36,38] In potential acute pulmonary edema, the acid-base balance is held in an alkaline status, which provides a buffer from acidosis precipitated by an acute deterioration. A prevailing respiratory alkalosis would cause a leftward shift of the oxygen dissociation curve, thereby assisting oxygen uptake within the lung. The large swings in pleural pressure, which are related to unobstructed hyperventilation, have the effect of attenuating sympathetic activity and entraining systemic blood pressure and heart rate.[39,56] However, the pleural pressure swings are transient (~50% of the cycle length) and less than those seen with OSA.[57] This entrainment effect on heart rate variability can be so profound that the patterns of heart rate variability that can develop are unique to CSA-CSR and contrast with OSA and HF with normal ventilation.[39] With prolonged exhalation and a closed upper airway, small amounts of intrinsic positive end-expiratory pressure may also develop, which could assist in preventing alveolar collapse. Large respiratory efforts also offset bronchoconstriction related to HF and edema.[58] Thus CSA-CSR may be a compensatory response to HF with subacute pulmonary edema.[58,59]

SUMMARY

CSA-CSR is a disorder characterized by cyclic hyperventilation with hypocapnia, triggered by the state change or arousal commonly seen in advanced HF of all causes. Snoring may occur during the peak of ventilation. The AHI is a crude marker of CSA-CSR severity and consideration should always be given to collateral history and examination, plus markers of cardiac and sleep dysfunction, plus quality of life when deciding whether to monitor or to manage. Loop gain (a ratio of ventilation to corresponding apnea) may be an alternative objective marker of CSA-CSR severity. Positive airway pressure is a treatment option that assists cardiac function and improves oxygen delivery, and is unique to CSA-CSR. In contrast, CPAP in OSA has its major role in upper airway stabilization, as indicated by a decrease in AHI to negligible levels.

REFERENCES

1. Bradley TD, McNicholas WT, Rutherford R, et al. Clinical and physiologic heterogeneity of the central sleep apnea syndrome. Am Rev Respir Dis 1986;134(2):217–21.
2. Sin DD, Fitzgerald F, Parker JD, et al. Risk factors for central and obstructive sleep apnea in 450 men and women with congestive heart failure. Am J Respir Crit Care Med 1999;160(4):1101–6.
3. Javaheri S, Parker TJ, Liming JD, et al. Sleep apnea in 81 ambulatory male patients with stable heart failure. Types and their prevalences, consequences, and presentations. Circulation 1998; 97(21):2154–9.
4. Solin P, Bergin P, Richardson M, et al. Influence of pulmonary capillary wedge pressure on central apnea in heart failure. Circulation 1999;99(12): 1574–9.
5. Pinna GD, Maestri R, Mortara A, et al. Pathophysiological and clinical relevance of simplified monitoring of nocturnal breathing disorders in heart failure patients. Eur J Heart Fail 2009; 11(3):264–72.
6. Naughton MT, Lorenzi-Filho G. Sleep in heart failure. Prog Cardiovasc Dis 2009;51(4):339–49.
7. Nopmaneejumruslers C, Kaneko Y, Hajek V, et al. Cheyne-Stokes respiration in stroke: relationship to hypocapnia and occult cardiac dysfunction. Am J Respir Crit Care Med 2005;171(9):1048–52.
8. Yumino D, Wang H, Floras JS, et al. Prevalence and physiological predictors of sleep apnea in patients with heart failure and systolic dysfunction. J Card Fail 2009;15(4):279–85.
9. Phillipson EA. Control of breathing during sleep. Am Rev Respir Dis 1978;118(5):909–39.
10. Phillipson EA, Bradley TD. Central sleep apnea. Clin Chest Med 1992;13(3):493–505.
11. Naughton M, Benard D, Tam A, et al. Role of hyperventilation in the pathogenesis of central sleep

apneas in patients with congestive heart failure. Am Rev Respir Dis 1993;148(2):330–8.

12. Hanly P, Zuberi N, Gray G. Pathogenesis of Cheyne-Stokes respiration in patients with congestive heart failure. Relationship to arterial PCO_2. Chest 1993;104:1079–84.

13. Tkacova R, Niroumand M, Lorenzi-Filho G, et al. Overnight shift from obstructive to central apneas in patients with heart failure: role of PCO_2 and circulatory delay. Circulation 2001;103(2):238–43.

14. Xie A, Skatrud JB, Puleo DS, et al. Apnea-hypopnea threshold for CO_2 in patients with congestive heart failure. Am J Respir Crit Care Med 2002;165(9):1245–50.

15. Nakayama H, Smith CA, Rodman JR, et al. Effect of ventilatory drive on carbon dioxide sensitivity below eupnea during sleep. Am J Respir Crit Care Med 2002;165(9):1251–60.

16. Sankri-Tarbichi AG, Grullon K, Badr MS. Effects of clonidine on breathing during sleep and susceptibility to central apnoea. Respir Physiol Neurobiol 2013;185(2):356–61.

17. Solin P, Roebuck T, Swieca J, et al. Effects of cardiac dysfunction on non-hypercapnic central sleep apnea. Chest 1998;113(1):104–10.

18. Hall MJ, Xie A, Rutherford R, et al. Cycle length of periodic breathing in patients with and without heart failure. Am J Respir Crit Care Med 1996;154(2 Pt 1):376–81.

19. Sands SA, Edwards BA, Kee K, et al. Loop gain as a means to predict a positive airway pressure suppression of Cheyne-Stokes respiration in patients with heart failure. Am J Respir Crit Care Med 2011;184(9):1067–75.

20. Khoo MC, Gottschalk A, Pack AI. Sleep-induced periodic breathing and apnea: a theoretical study. J Appl Physiol 1991;70(5):2014–24.

21. Solin P, Roebuck T, Johns DP, et al. Peripheral and central ventilatory responses in central sleep apnea with and without congestive heart failure. Am J Respir Crit Care Med 2000;162(6):2194–200.

22. Szollosi I, Thompson BR, Krum H, et al. Impaired pulmonary diffusing capacity and hypoxia in heart failure correlates with central sleep apnea severity. Chest 2008;134(1):67–72.

23. Churchill ED, Cope O. The rapid shallow breathing resulting from pulmonary congestion and edema. J Exp Med 1929;49(4):531–7.

24. Lorenzi-Filho G, Azevedo ER, Parker JD, et al. Relationship of carbon dioxide tension in arterial blood to pulmonary wedge pressure in heart failure. Eur Respir J 2002;19(1):37–40.

25. Mansfield DR, Solin P, Roebuck T, et al. The effect of successful heart transplant treatment of heart failure on central sleep apnea. Chest 2003;124(5):1675–81.

26. Yumino D, Redolfi S, Ruttanaumpawan P, et al. Nocturnal rostral fluid shift: a unifying concept for the pathogenesis of obstructive and central sleep apnea in men with heart failure. Circulation 2010;121(14):1598–605.

27. Solin P, Snell GI, Williams TJ, et al. Central sleep apnoea in congestive heart failure despite vagal denervation after bilateral lung transplantation. Eur Respir J 1998;12(2):495–8.

28. Sun SY, Wang W, Zucker IH, et al. Enhanced activity of carotid body chemoreceptors in rabbits with heart failure: role of nitric oxide. J Appl Physiol 1999;86(4):1273–82.

29. Naughton MT, Benard DC, Liu PP, et al. Effects of nasal CPAP on sympathetic activity in patients with heart failure and central sleep apnea. Am J Respir Crit Care Med 1995;152(2):473–9.

30. Solin P, Kaye DM, Little PJ, et al. Impact of sleep apnea on sympathetic nervous system activity in heart failure. Chest 2003;123(4):1119–26.

31. Mansfield D, Kaye DM, Brunner La Rocca H, et al. Raised sympathetic nerve activity in heart failure and central sleep apnea is due to heart failure severity. Circulation 2003;107(10):1396–400.

32. Badr MS, Toiber F, Skatrud JB, et al. Pharyngeal narrowing/occlusion during central sleep apnea. J Appl Physiol 1995;78(5):1806–15.

33. Alex CG, Onal E, Lopata M. Upper airway occlusion during sleep in patients with Cheyne-Stokes respiration. Am Rev Respir Dis 1986;133(1):42–5.

34. Niinimaa V, Cole P, Mintz S, et al. The switching point from nasal to oronasal breathing. Respir Physiol 1980;42(1):61–71.

35. Niinimaa V, Cole P, Mintz S, et al. Oronasal distribution of respiratory airflow. Respir Physiol 1981;43(1):69–75.

36. Yumino D, Kasai T, Kimmerly D, et al. Differing effects of obstructive and central sleep apneas on stroke volume in patients with heart failure. Am J Respir Crit Care Med 2013;187(4):433–8.

37. Parker JD, Brooks D, Kozar LF, et al. Acute and chronic effects of airway obstruction on canine left ventricular performance. Am J Respir Crit Care Med 1999;160(6):1888–96.

38. Maze SS, Kotler MN, Parry WR. Doppler evaluation of changing cardiac dynamics during Cheyne-Stokes respiration. Chest 1989;95(3):525–9.

39. Szollosi I, Krum H, Kaye D, et al. Sleep apnea in heart failure increases heart rate variability and sympathetic dominance. Sleep 2007;30(11):1509–14.

40. Kee K, Naughton MT. Heart failure and the lung. Circ J 2010;74(12):2507–16.

41. Brack T, Jubran A, Tobin MJ. Dyspnea and decreased variability of breathing in patients with restrictive lung disease. Am J Respir Crit Care Med 2002;165(9):1260–4.

42. Lorenzi-Filho G, Rankin F, Bies I, et al. Effects of inhaled carbon dioxide and oxygen on Cheyne-Stokes respiration in patients with heart failure. Am J Respir Crit Care Med 1999;159(5 Pt 1): 1490–8.

43. Altschule MD, Iglauer A. The effect of position on periodic breathing in chronic cardiac decompensation. N Engl J Med 1958;259(22):1064–6.

44. Sahlin C, Svanborg E, Stenlund H, et al. Cheyne-Stokes respiration and supine dependency. Eur Respir J 2005;25(5):829–33.

45. Leung RS, Bowman ME, Parker JD, et al. Avoidance of the left lateral decubitus position during sleep in patients with heart failure: relationship to cardiac size and function. J Am Coll Cardiol 2003;41(2):227–30.

46. Szollosi I, Roebuck T, Thompson B, et al. Lateral sleeping position reduces severity of central sleep apnea/Cheyne-Stokes respiration. Sleep 2006; 29(8):1045–51.

47. Hurewitz AN, Susskind H, Harold WH. Obesity alters regional ventilation in lateral decubitus position. J Appl Physiol 1985;59(3):774–83.

48. Pump B, Videbaek R, Gabrielsen A, et al. Arterial pressure in humans during weightlessness induced by parabolic flights. J Appl Physiol 1999;87(3):928–32.

49. Arzt M, Young T, Finn L, et al. Sleepiness and sleep in patients with both systolic heart failure and obstructive sleep apnea. Arch Intern Med 2006; 166(16):1716–22.

50. Hanly P, Zuberi N. Periodic leg movements during sleep before and after heart transplantation. Sleep 1992;15(6):489–92.

51. Solin P, Jackson DM, Roebuck T, et al. Cardiac diastolic function and hypercapnic ventilatory responses in central sleep apnoea. Eur Respir J 2002;20(3):717–23.

52. Series F, Kimoff RJ, Morrison D, et al. Prospective evaluation of nocturnal oximetry for detection of sleep-related breathing disturbances in patients with chronic heart failure. Chest 2005;127(5): 1507–14.

53. Weinreich G, Armitstead J, Topfer V, et al. Validation of ApneaLink as screening device for Cheyne-Stokes respiration. Sleep 2009;32(4): 553–7.

54. Berry RB, Budhiraja R, Gottlieb DJ, et al. Rules for scoring respiratory events in sleep: update of the 2007 AASM Manual for the Scoring of Sleep and Associated Events. Deliberations of the Sleep Apnea Definitions Task Force of the American Academy of Sleep Medicine. J Clin Sleep Med 2012; 8(5):597–619.

55. Naughton MT. Loop gain in apnea: gaining control or controlling the gain? Am J Respir Crit Care Med 2010;181(2):103–5.

56. Lorenzi-Filho G, Dajani HR, Leung RS, et al. Entrainment of blood pressure and heart rate oscillations by periodic breathing. Am J Respir Crit Care Med 1999;159(4 Pt 1):1147–54.

57. Suzuki M, Ogawa H, Okabe S, et al. Digital recording and analysis of esophageal pressure for patients with obstructive sleep apnea-hypopnea syndrome. Sleep Breath 2005;9(2): 64–72.

58. Naughton MT. Cheyne-Stokes respiration: friend or foe? Thorax 2012;67(4):357–60.

59. Naughton MT. Is Cheyne-Stokes respiration detrimental in patients with heart failure? Sleep Breath 2000;4(3):127–8.

Central Sleep Apnea and Cardiovascular Disease

Sean M. Caples, DO

KEYWORDS

- Central sleep apnea • Heart failure • Cheyne-Stokes respiration • Cardiovascular disease

KEY POINTS

- Central sleep apnea (CSA) is thought to occur as a consequence of heart failure (HF), with a prevalence estimated at 1 in 3.
- Some evidence suggests that the presence of CSA worsens the prognosis and outcomes in HF.
- The optimization of medical management should be the first step in the management of CSA in HF.
- Positive airway pressure devices, such as adaptive servo-ventilation, are effective at controlling CSA, but the results of large clinical trials are awaited to determine whether the targeted treatment of CSA improves important outcomes in HF.
- Atrial fibrillation (AF) seems to be a risk factor for CSA in HF populations, but CSA is also commonly encountered in AF without left ventricular dysfunction.

EPIDEMIOLOGY: HEART FAILURE

Because of the varied definitions and tools to define and measure heart failure (HF), precise estimates of its epidemiology are lacking. In general, HF may be subclassified into left ventricular (LV) systolic dysfunction, whereby there are measurable reductions in contractility, and LV diastolic dysfunction, also known as HF with preserved ejection fraction. The proportion of HF attributed to diastolic dysfunction may be as high as 50%.[1,2] Furthermore, it is estimated that as many as half of the people in the community with measurable LV dysfunction are asymptomatic.

HF is a public health problem, with most recent estimates of more than 5 million individuals in the United States afflicted.[3] With an aging population, the incidence of HF continues to increase, with now greater than 500,000 new cases per year. Over the course of a lifetime, one's risk for HF approaches 20%.[4] Despite the development of increasingly sophisticated drug and device therapies, mortality rates related to HF remain high. It is among these reasons that there is an intense interest in the interplay between HF and central sleep apnea (CSA) in the hopes of better understanding pathophysiologic mechanisms and building a greater armamentarium of treatments to combat HF.

EPIDEMIOLOGY: CSA IN HF

There are similar imprecisions in determining the epidemiology of CSA in HF. For the most part, existing literature is composed of small case series, which generally originate from sleep laboratory referral populations. The range of CSA in HF reported in these studies range from 15% to 30%.[5–8] Such studies, also influenced by participatory bias, may overestimate the true occurrence of CSA in those with HF. On the other hand, accounting for the substantial proportion of those in the community with asymptomatic LV dysfunction, it is just as possible that the true prevalence of CSA is underestimated.

Because efforts to establish a causal relationship between CSA and important outcomes in HF rely in part on an accurate accounting of the burden of CSA in the HF population, other limitations to the existing epidemiologic literature are

Division of Pulmonary and Critical Care Medicine, Center for Sleep Medicine, Mayo Clinic, 200 First Street SW, Rochester, MN 55905, USA
E-mail address: Caples.Sean@mayo.edu

Sleep Med Clin 9 (2014) 27–35
http://dx.doi.org/10.1016/j.jsmc.2013.10.007
1556-407X/14/$ – see front matter © 2014 Elsevier Inc. All rights reserved.

worth mentioning. First, it is important to recognize that patients with HF also have a high rate of obstructive sleep apnea (OSA), often in combination with CSA.[8] This coupling likely represents an overlap of the pathophysiologic and neuromuscular mechanisms that govern aspects of both ventilatory control and upper airway patency. Traditionally, prevalence studies in HF, rather than focusing purely on CSA, have reported rates of *sleep-disordered breathing* (SDB), encompassing both OSA and CSA. Rates of SDB in these series have been reported as high as 50% to 60%. In such instances, it is difficult to disentangle the effects of CSA in patients with HF from those caused by OSA. In speaking to the differential effects of OSA and CSA in HF, there is an overnight shift in predominance of obstructive apneas early in the sleep period to central apneas later on, an effect that may be mediated by deteriorating cardiac function attributable to obstructive breathing events.[9]

Second, there are shortcomings to the use of the apnea-hypopnea index (AHI) in quantifying the severity of CSA and, therefore, in determining a dose-response effect of CSA on cardiovascular outcomes. By convention and ease of application, but without sound evidence for validation, clinicians and researchers traditionally apply the AHI to CSA as they would to OSA. Although the AHI has been well established to correlate with outcomes in OSA, similar validation data do not exist in the setting of CSA, as outlined in the American Academy of Sleep Medicine's scoring manual.[10] Various metrics are scattered in the literature, including the central apnea index[11]; the central AHI; sleep time spent with an oxyhemoglobin saturation of less than 90%; and the Cheyne-Stokes respiration (CSR) time, which measures the proportion of sleep time with periodic breathing.[7,12] One study found prognostic significance in the central AHI but not in the percentage of sleep time spent with periodic breathing.[12] Future standardization will be needed to help better delineate the relationship between CSA and cardiovascular outcomes.

Finally, important temporal trends in the management of HF may confound the relationship between CSA and HF. Because CSA is generally thought to occur as a consequence of HF, the first approach to treatment is medical optimization of HF, which, as discussed later, attenuates CSA. The paradigm shift to include β-blockers as the standard therapy for HF gained traction in the late 1990s,[13] a period *after* most of the existing epidemiologic literature on CSA and HF was established. A suggestion was made by the investigators of the Canadian Continuous Positive Airway Pressure for Patients with Central Sleep Apnea and Heart Failure Trial (CANPAP), a large randomized controlled trial of continuous positive airway pressure (CPAP) therapy in CSA and HF, that such medical treatments of HF substantially reduced the rates of CSA in HF, to the point that recruitment to the trial was fatally wounded,[14] and that more contemporary analyses would prove that CSA has become less common over time. However, a more recent ascertainment of sleep apnea in consecutive patients with HF, all of whom were treated with β-blockers, showed a historically similar prevalence of CSA (31%).[7]

CLINICAL IMPLICATIONS OF CSA IN HF

There are important signs and symptoms seen in patients with HF that may directly link to CSA. The cycles of apnea and hyperpnea characteristic of CSA-CSR can result in the paroxysmal nocturnal dyspnea classically associated with HF. CSA-CSR tends to be augmented by the supine position,[15] which may contribute to the classic HF symptom of orthopnea. Finally, in CSA-CSR, sleep is studded with arousals that tend to occur at the height of the hyperpneic phase.[16] By virtue of the typical CSA-CSR cycle length, these arousals often number in excess of 40 per hour. With few exceptions,[17] studies specifically measuring sleep-related complaints in patients with pure CSA are lacking; but there is a notable lack of such symptoms in community-based HF samples with a high rate of severe OSA.[18]

Rather than these uncommonly reported symptoms, sleep and nonsleep clinicians remain focused on whether or not the presence of CSA is detrimental to important cardiovascular outcomes in patients with HF, such as mortality and HF exacerbations. Proof of the concept comes from observations of repeated hypoxemia, evidence for sympatho-excitation, and sleep fragmentation in fragile patients with compromised cardiac function. The finding of CSA in patients with asymptomatic LV dysfunction, independent of hemodynamic measures, suggests that CSA may precede the development of and, therefore, pose a risk factor for overt HF.[19]

Despite what may seem like an intuitive relationship, available small studies have been conflicting in their conclusions. CSA-CSR in HF has been associated with increased mortality in some studies,[12,20] with multivariate analysis suggesting that CSA-CSR may be an independent risk factor for mortality.[12,21] However, one of the largest studies to date, of patients with HF referred for cardiac transplantation, did not find an effect of CSA on long-term outcomes.[22] It is worth mentioning that there is significant heterogeneity in the available studies in terms of patient baseline characteristics (age, criteria for the diagnosis of CSA by AHI, presence of arrhythmias) and the fact that CSA was sometimes treated in noncontrolled settings (**Table 1**).[23] Finally, further attesting to the link between CSA and the severity of HF, those with CSA-CSR during wakefulness or exercise have worse outcomes.

TREATMENT OF CSA

Treatment of CSA in patients with HF with sleep-related symptoms, such as daytime sleepiness or repetitive awakenings, seems warranted.[24] However, as noted earlier, such complaints are uncommon in HF populations, which raises the important question of whether or not otherwise asymptomatic patients with HF found to have CSA should be treated because of the potential for cardiovascular benefit. Similar questions have been asked about patients with OSA with comorbid cardiovascular disease where there is considerable observational and interventional published data but no clear answers. In the setting of CSA, there is even less guidance, though clinical opinion and sentiment are strong.

MEDICAL OPTIMIZATION: PHARMACOLOGIC INTERVENTION

The first intervention in patients with CSA and HF should be medical optimization.[25] In general, this involves pharmacologic therapy, which, among other mechanisms, improves hemodynamics and reduces cardiac filling pressures. Angiotensin-converting enzyme inhibitors[26] and β-blockers[27] attenuate CSA in HF. Acute diuretic therapy was found to improve sleep apnea in patients with volume overload and diastolic dysfunction.[28] Not all cases of medical optimization are effective; one study showed attenuation of breathing events in a minority of patients after 2 months of medical therapy following acute HF.[29]

MEDICAL OPTIMIZATION: SURGERY/DEVICES/CARDIAC PACING

Beyond drug therapy, there is further evidence that invasive treatments for HF resulting in improvements in cardiac function will often have concordant improvements in CSA. Notably, such treatments are indicated as primary therapy for HF and are not recommended as first-line CSA treatment. Case reports of surgical correction of mitral valvular disease for HF management describe marked improvement in CSA-CSR.[30] Cardiac transplantation in severe HF resulted in eradication of

CSA-CSR in 7 of 13 patients, although for reasons that are not clear, disordered breathing persisted in another 4 patients postoperatively.[31]

A high-profile publication suggesting an improvement in OSA by atrial overdrive pacing[32] was subsequently disproved by several larger, more rigorously conducted studies.[33] However, closer examination of the initial study results showed subtle reductions in recorded central apneas, suggesting that increases in cardiac output, with reduced circulation time, may enhance ventilatory stability in HF. Along the same lines, cardiac resynchronization therapy (CRT), also known as biventricular pacing, may hold promise in treating CSA in patients with HF with ventricular conduction delay. CRT has been shown to significantly decrease the number of apneas, increase oxygen saturation, and improve sleep quality in such patients.[34] Although seductive to consider, it is yet to be proven whether some of the survival benefit attributed to CRT in patients with HF in large-scale studies[35,36] may be related to the amelioration of central apnea in this population.

Finally, there are recent reports of the use of phrenic nerve stimulation (PNS) by an implanted transvenous device in patients with HF and CSA. One night of unilateral PNS improved some indices of CSA and was not associated with significant adverse events.[37] These patients had a high rate of HF related to rheumatic fever, and many were not on standard medical therapy. Much more research is needed to learn whether invasive treatments such as these are warranted in specific populations and whether any benefit is derived over and above that related to enhancing cardiac function.

POSITIVE AIRWAY PRESSURE
CPAP

Independent of its effects on the upper airway and ventilation, CPAP has salutary effects on cardiac function in HF on account of inspiratory muscle unloading and reduction of cardiac preload and afterload related to increasing intrathoracic pressure.[38] A small controlled trial of CPAP or usual care followed those with HF with and without CSA. CPAP was associated with an increase in ejection fraction and reduced risk of heart transplant only in those with CSA.[39] Another trial of CPAP in HF with CSA showed reductions in catecholamine levels.[40]

The multicenter CANPAP Trial randomized patients with systolic HF and CSA to CPAP or no CPAP.[14] Although the trial showed small improvements in CSA, ejection fraction, and sympathetic activity in the CPAP group, it failed to show

Table 1
Available observational studies describing outcomes in patients with HF with CSA

	Lanfranchi et al,[12] 1999	Sin et al,[39] 2000	Corra et al,[61] 2006	Javaheri et al,[21] 2007	Brack et al,[62] 2007	Roebuck et al,[22] 2004	Luo et al,[63] 2010
Patients (n)	62	66	133	88	60	78	128
Outcome	Death, Tx	Death, Tx	Death, Tx	Death	Death, Tx	Death	Death
Risk associated with CSR[a]	+	+ 2.53	+ 5.7	+ 2.1	(+) 3.8	—	—
AHI defining presence of CSR cycles per hour	≥30	≥15	>30	≥5	≥15	>5	≥5
LVEF (%)	23	22	23	24	26	20	36
Mean observation period (y)	2.3	2.2	3.2	4.3	2.3	4.3	2.9
Remarks	Patients, with AF excluded	CSR treated	CSR during exercise and sleep	CSR treated	CSR during daytime	CSR treated	—

Abbreviations: AF, atrial fibrillation; LVEF, left ventricular ejection fraction; Tx, survival without cardiac transplantation.

[a] Hazard ratio controlled for several confounders, with + and − denoting increased mortality and equal mortality of CSR versus no CSR, respectively.

Data from Brack T, Randerath W, Bloch KE. Cheyne-Stokes respiration in patients with heart failure: prevalence, causes, consequences and treatments. Respiration 2012;83(2):168.

a benefit in the primary outcome, transplant-free survival. In fact, an interim analysis after a mean follow-up of 24 months suggested a trend toward greater mortality in the CPAP group, a finding that eventually dissipated with further observation. As noted earlier, the investigators hypothesized that improvements in medical therapy over the course of the multi-year study (use of β-blockers in particular) reduced mortality in all patients to the point of irreversibly underpowering the study. In fact, death rates in both groups were considerably less than predicted in the power analysis. That said, it is noteworthy that the overall AHI was reduced by only about 50% in the CPAP group, and, as in many trials of CPAP, adherence to therapy was suboptimal. Yet, in a post hoc analysis of CANPAP, in those patients whom CPAP effectively suppressed CSA-CSR, LV ejection fraction (LVEF) and transplant-free survival were improved compared with controls, suggesting CPAP may be an effective therapy in selected individuals **(Fig. 1)**.[41]

Adaptive Servo-Ventilation

Adaptive servo-ventilation (ASV) uses an algorithm to analyze a patient's ventilation and then adjusts pressure support to reach a calculated ventilation target. The algorithms by which the devices accomplish this are proprietary, and no comparative efficacy trials have been published to guide the selection of various machines that are available in the marketplace.

Although providing support during apneas and hypopneas, ASV is designed to avoid overventilation during the hyperpneic phase, promoting more uniform ventilation and reducing arousals from sleep. Available within the United States since 2006, ASV has been shown to effectively suppress CSA-CSR; improve LVEF, quality of life,[42] and exercise capacity[43]; and may be preferred over CPAP by patients.[11,44,45] A 1-month randomized trial comparing therapeutic ASV with subtherapeutic ASV showed significant improvements in daytime sleepiness and reductions in neurohormonal activity associated with active treatment in patients with stable HF and CSR-CSA.[46] A recent systematic review and meta-analysis identified 14 studies comparing ASV with control conditions, defined as other positive airway pressure (PAP) modes (including CPAP and bilevel PAP), oxygen therapy subtherapeutic ASV, or no treatment.[47] The investigators concluded that ASV was more effective than control conditions in reducing the AHI and improving cardiac function and exercise capacity. Based on these encouraging preliminary data, large multicenter trials are now underway to determine if ASV will impact important cardiovascular outcomes, such as mortality, on a larger scale.[48]

Nocturnal Gas (Oxygen and Carbon Dioxide) Supplementation

Supplemental oxygen as treatment of CSA is thought to suppress ventilatory drive,[49] thereby

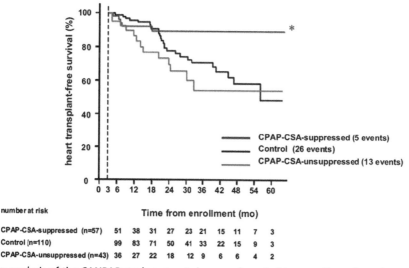

number at risk

CPAP-CSA-suppressed (n=57)	51	38	31	27	23	21	15	11	7	3
Control (n=110)		99	83	71	50	41	33	22	15	9	3
CPAP-CSA-unsuppressed (n=43)	36	27	22	18		12	9	6	6	4	2

Fig. 1. Post hoc analysis of the CANPAP study suggests improved survival in a small number of patients in whom CPAP effectively suppressed CSA. * denotes P<.05. (*From* Arzt M, Floras JS, Logan AG, et al. Suppression of central sleep apnea by continuous positive airway pressure and transplant-free survival in heart failure: a post hoc analysis of the Canadian Continuous Positive Airway Pressure for Patients with Central Sleep Apnea and Heart Failure Trial (CANPAP). Circulation 2007;115(25):3178; with permission.)

buffering the apneic threshold; but it is also possible that oxygen improves cardiac function, thereby indirectly reducing CSA. A small, 2-night, randomized controlled trial yielded a reduced AHI in men with severe HF and nocturnal hypoxemia[50]; there is evidence for improved quality of life and exercise capacity associated with oxygen therapy in HF. As in device therapy discussed earlier, whether such improvements are directly attributable to attenuation of CSA remains speculative.

Because hypocapnia seems to be intimately related to the pathogenesis of CSA-CSR, it would follow that increasing $Paco_2$ by the inhalation of carbon dioxide (CO_2) or by increasing dead space may ameliorate ventilatory instability characteristic of the breathing disorder. One night of inhaled CO_2 administered to 6 patients with severe stable HF resulted in virtual eradication of CSA-CSR.[51] However, longer-term studies are lacking; there is evidence for worsened sleep quality and fragmented sleep architecture associated with CO_2 treatment. Moreover, the finding of an increase in sympathetic activity after a single night of CO_2 treatment may be harmful in those with HF.[52]

NOVEL DRUG THERAPY
Theophylline

Theophylline, a phosphodiesterase inhibitor with bronchodilatory properties, has been shown to be a central respiratory stimulant,[53] possibly by antagonizing adenosine in the brainstem. Historically, use of theophylline has fallen out of favor because of the risk of neuro-excitatory effects, such as tachycardia, which are typically coupled to serum concentrations more than the therapeutic range of 10 to 20 μg/mL. In a controlled trial of 15 men with stable congestive heart failure (LVEF <45%), 5 days of oral theophylline, resulting in modest serum concentrations (11 μg/mL), reduced the frequency of central apneas and hypopneas as well as the duration of arterial oxyhemoglobin desaturation.[54] Safety concerns related to the risk of arrhythmogenesis in patients with HF, a population with sympathetic overactivity, may be tempered by a subsequent study that showed similarly modest serum theophylline levels do not increase sympathetic activity or heart rate in patients with HF as they do in healthy individuals.[55] Nevertheless, caution is warranted because the long-term use of another oral phosphodiesterase inhibitor, milrinone, was shown to actually increase mortality in patients with HF.[56]

Acetazolamide

Acetazolamide, a carbonic anhydrase inhibitor, has 2 effects that may be beneficial in the setting of CSA and HF. First, diuretic effects reduce pulmonary congestion. Second, it induces a metabolic acidosis to stimulate respiration. In a randomized placebo controlled trial of 6 nights of single-dose acetazolamide in a small group of men with stable HF and CSA, acetazolamide significantly improved the central apnea index (mean 44 to 23 per hour) as well as the nadir oxygen saturation value compared with placebo.[57] That the $Paco_2$ was found to be lower in the treatment group confirms the importance of the *difference* between the prevailing $Paco_2$ and the $Paco_2$ associated with the apneic threshold, rather than the absolute values, in triggering ventilatory instability.

CSA and Atrial Fibrillation

Because it is the most common arrhythmia encountered in clinical practice and is associated with serious conditions, such as stroke, HF, and mortality,[58] there is increasing interest in the relationship between atrial fibrillation (AF) and sleep apnea syndromes. Most of the focus has been on AF and OSA because the sequelae of obstructive apneas, particularly sympathetic surges and swings in intrathoracic pressure, are a neat pathophysiologic fit to explain the alterations in the electrical properties of the thin-walled atria there is ongoing interest in whether PAP therapy for OSA may alter important outcomes.

However, there is also evidence for a link between AF and CSA. On the one hand, the presence of LV dysfunction or overt HF may mediate (if not confound) the relationship because AF and HF frequently coexist. Sin and colleagues,[8] in their polysomnographic assessment of 450 men and women with HF, found AF to be more tightly associated with CSA than OSA. A recent case report provides evidence for a bidirectional relationship between CSA and AF, with the onset of CSA following a paroxysm of AF, presumably because of acute deterioration in cardiac function associated with arrhythmia onset.[59]

On the other hand, evidence arguing against the prerequisite of LV dysfunction in the interaction between AF and CSA comes from Leung and colleagues,[60] who showed a high prevalence of AF in those with idiopathic CSA and free of overt HF. Further research is needed to better explain this relationship and, in the absence of any interventional trials, whether the treatment of CSA impacts measurable outcomes in AF.

REFERENCES

1. Owan TE, Hodge DO, Herges RM, et al. Trends in prevalence and outcome of heart failure with

preserved ejection fraction. N Engl J Med 2006; 355(3):251–9.

2. Bursi F, Weston SA, Redfield MM, et al. Systolic and diastolic heart failure in the community. JAMA 2006;296(18):2209–16.

3. Go AS, Mozaffarian D, Roger VL, et al. Executive summary: heart disease and stroke statistics– 2013 update: a report from the American Heart Association. Circulation 2013;127(1):143–52.

4. Lloyd-Jones DM, Larson MG, Leip EP, et al. Life-time risk for developing congestive heart failure: the Framingham Heart Study. Circulation 2002; 106(24):3068–72.

5. Yumino D, Wang H, Floras JS, et al. Prevalence and physiological predictors of sleep apnea in pa-tients with heart failure and systolic dysfunction. J Card Fail 2009;15(4):279–85.

6. Ferrier K, Campbell A, Yee B, et al. Sleep-disor-dered breathing occurs frequently in stable outpa-tients with congestive heart failure. Chest 2005; 128(4):2116–22.

7. MacDonald M, Fang J, Pittman SD, et al. The cur-rent prevalence of sleep disordered breathing in congestive heart failure patients treated with beta-blockers. J Clin Sleep Med 2008;4(1):38–42.

8. Sin DD, Fitzgerald F, Parker JD, et al. Risk factors for central and obstructive sleep apnea in 450 men and women with congestive heart failure. Am J Respir Crit Care Med 1999;160(4):1101–6.

9. Tkacova R, Niroumand M, Lorenzi-Filho G, et al. Overnight shift from obstructive to central apneas in patients with heart failure: role of PCO2 and cir-culatory delay. Circulation 2001;103(2):238–43.

10. Redline S, Budhiraja R, Kapur V, et al. The scoring of respiratory events in sleep: reliability and validity. J Clin Sleep Med 2007;3(2):169–200.

11. Teschler H, Dohring J, Wang YM, et al. Adaptive pressure support servo-ventilation: a novel treat-ment for Cheyne-Stokes respiration in heart failure. Am J Respir Crit Care Med 2001;164(4):614–9.

12. Lanfranchi PA, Braghiroli A, Bosimini E, et al. Prog-nostic value of nocturnal Cheyne-Stokes respira-tion in chronic heart failure. Circulation 1999; 99(11):1435–40.

13. Foody JM, Farrell MH, Krumholz HM. Beta-blocker therapy in heart failure: scientific review. JAMA 2002;287(7):883–9.

14. Bradley TD, Logan AG, Kimoff RJ, et al. Continuous positive airway pressure for central sleep apnea and heart failure. N Engl J Med 2005;353(19): 2025–33.

15. Sahlin C, Svanborg E, Stenlund H, et al. Cheyne-Stokes respiration and supine dependency. Eur Respir J 2005;25(5):829–33.

16. Eckert DJ, Jordan AS, Merchia P, et al. Central sleep apnea: pathophysiology and treatment. Chest 2007;131(2):595–607.

17. Staniforth AD, Kinnear WJ, Starling R, et al. Effect of oxygen on sleep quality, cognitive func-tion and sympathetic activity in patients with chronic heart failure and Cheyne-Stokes respira-tion. Eur Heart J 1998;19(6):922–8.

18. Arzt M, Young T, Finn L, et al. Sleepiness and sleep in patients with both systolic heart failure and obstructive sleep apnea. Arch Intern Med 2006; 166(16):1716–22.

19. Lanfranchi PA, Somers VK, Braghiroli A, et al. Central sleep apnea in left ventricular dysfunction: preva-lence and implications for arrhythmic risk. Circulation 2003;107(5):727–32.

20. Hanly P, Zuberi-Khokhar N. Increased mortality associated with Cheyne-Stokes respiration in pa-tients with congestive heart failure. Am J Respir Crit Care Med 1996;153(1):272–6.

21. Javaheri S, Shukla R, Zeigler H, et al. Central sleep apnea, right ventricular dysfunction, and low dia-stolic blood pressure are predictors of mortality in systolic heart failure. J Am Coll Cardiol 2007; 49(20):2028–34.

22. Roebuck T, Solin P, Kaye DM, et al. Increased long-term mortality in heart failure due to sleep apnoea is not yet proven. Eur Respir J 2004;23(5):735–40.

23. Brack T, Randerath W, Bloch KE. Cheyne-Stokes respiration in patients with heart failure: preva-lence, causes, consequences and treatments. Respiration 2012;83(2):165–76.

24. Aurora RN, Chowdhuri S, Ramar K, et al. The treat-ment of central sleep apnea syndromes in adults: practice parameters with an evidence-based litera-ture review and meta-analyses. Sleep 2012;35(1): 17–40.

25. Jessup M, Abraham WT, Casey DE, et al. 2009 focused update: ACCF/AHA guidelines for the diag-nosis and management of heart failure in adults: a report of the American College of Cardiology Foun-dation/American Heart Association Task Force on practice guidelines: developed in collaboration with the International Society for Heart and Lung Trans-plantation. Circulation 2009;119(14):1977–2016.

26. Walsh JT, Andrews R, Starling R, et al. Effects of captopril and oxygen on sleep apnoea in patients with mild to moderate congestive cardiac failure. Br Heart J 1995;73(3):237–41.

27. Tamura A, Kawano Y, Kadota J. Carvedilol reduces the severity of central sleep apnea in chronic heart failure. Circ J 2009;73(2):295–8.

28. Bucca CB, Brussino L, Battisti A, et al. Diuretics in obstructive sleep apnea with diastolic heart failure. Chest 2007;132(2):440–6.

29. Tremel F, Pepin JL, Veale D, et al. High prevalence and persistence of sleep apnoea in patients referred for acute left ventricular failure and medi-cally treated over 2 months. Eur Heart J 1999; 20(16):1201–9.

30. Rubin AE, Gottlieb SH, Gold AR, et al. Elimination of central sleep apnoea by mitral valvuloplasty: the role of feedback delay in periodic breathing. Thorax 2004;59(2):174–6.

31. Mansfield DR, Solin P, Roebuck T, et al. The effect of successful heart transplant treatment of heart failure on central sleep apnea. Chest 2003; 124(5):1675–81.

32. Garrigue S, Bordier P, Jais P, et al. Benefit of atrial pacing in sleep apnea syndrome. N Engl J Med 2002;346(6):404–12.

33. Luthje L, Unterberg-Buchwald C, Dajani D, et al. Atrial overdrive pacing in patients with sleep apnea with implanted pacemaker. Am J Respir Crit Care Med 2005;172(1):118–22.

34. Sinha AM, Skobel EC, Breithardt OA, et al. Cardiac resynchronization therapy improves central sleep apnea and Cheyne-Stokes respiration in patients with chronic heart failure. J Am Coll Cardiol 2004; 44(1):68–71.

35. Bristow MR, Saxon LA, Boehmer J, et al. Cardiac-resynchronization therapy with or without an implantable defibrillator in advanced chronic heart failure. N Engl J Med 2004;350(21):2140–50.

36. Cleland JG, Daubert J-C, Erdmann E, et al. The effect of cardiac resynchronization on morbidity and mortality in heart failure. N Engl J Med 2005; 352(15):1539–49.

37. Zhang XL, Ding N, Wang H, et al. Transvenous phrenic nerve stimulation in patients with Cheyne-Stokes respiration and congestive heart failure: a safety and proof-of-concept study. Chest 2012; 142(4):927–34.

38. Naughton MT, Rahman MA, Hara K, et al. Effect of continuous positive airway pressure on intrathoracic and left ventricular transmural pressures in patients with congestive heart failure. Circulation 1995;91(6):1725–31.

39. Sin DD, Logan AG, Fitzgerald FS, et al. Effects of continuous positive airway pressure on cardiovascular outcomes in heart failure patients with and without Cheyne-Stokes respiration. Circulation 2000;102(1):61–6.

40. Naughton M, Liu P, Bernard D, et al. Treatment of congestive heart failure and Cheyne-Stokes respiration during sleep by continuous positive airway pressure. Am J Respir Crit Care Med 1995; 151(1):92–7.

41. Arzt M, Floras JS, Logan AG, et al. Suppression of central sleep apnea by continuous positive airway pressure and transplant-free survival in heart failure: a post hoc analysis of the Canadian continuous positive airway pressure for patients with central sleep apnea and heart failure trial (CANPAP). Circulation 2007;115(25):3173–80.

42. Kasai T, Usui Y, Yoshioka T, et al. Effect of flow-triggered adaptive servo-ventilation compared with continuous positive airway pressure in patients with chronic heart failure with coexisting obstructive sleep apnea and Cheyne-Stokes respiration. Circ Heart Fail 2010;3(1):140–8.

43. Oldenburg O, Bitter T, Lehmann R, et al. Adaptive servoventilation improves cardiac function and respiratory stability. Clin Res Cardiol 2011;100(2): 107–15.

44. Philippe C, Stoica-Herman M, Drouot X, et al. Compliance with and effectiveness of adaptive servoventilation versus continuous positive airway pressure in the treatment of Cheyne-Stokes respiration in heart failure over a six month period. Heart 2006;92(3):337–42.

45. Morgenthaler TI, Gay PC, Gordon N, et al. Adaptive servoventilation versus noninvasive positive pressure ventilation for central, mixed, and complex sleep apnea syndromes. Sleep 2007;30(4):468–75.

46. Pepperell JC, Maskell NA, Jones DR, et al. A randomized controlled trial of adaptive ventilation for Cheyne-Stokes breathing in heart failure. Am J Respir Crit Care Med 2003;168(9):1109–14.

47. Sharma BK, Bakker JP, McSharry DG, et al. Adaptive servoventilation for treatment of sleep-disordered breathing in heart failure: a systematic review and meta-analysis. Chest 2012;142(5): 1211–21.

48. Cowie MR, Woehrle H, Wegscheider K, et al. Rationale and design of the SERVE-HF study: treatment of sleep-disordered breathing with predominant central sleep apnoea with adaptive servo-ventilation in patients with chronic heart failure. Eur J Heart Fail 2013;15(8):937–43.

49. Andreas S, von zur Muhlen F, Stevens J, et al. Nocturnal oxygen and hypercapnic ventilatory response in patients with congestive heart failure. Respir Med 1998;92(3):426–31.

50. Hanly PJ, Millar TW, Steljes DG, et al. The effect of oxygen on respiration and sleep in patients with congestive heart failure. Ann Intern Med 1989; 111(10):777–82.

51. Steens RD, Millar TW, Su X, et al. Effect of inhaled 3% CO_2 on Cheyne-Stokes respiration in congestive heart failure. Sleep 1994;17(1):61–8.

52. Andreas S, Weidel K, Hagenah G, et al. Treatment of Cheyne-Stokes respiration with nasal oxygen and carbon dioxide. Eur Respir J 1998;12(2):414–9.

53. Eldridge FL, Millhorn DE, Kiley JP. Antagonism by theophylline of respiratory inhibition induced by adenosine. J Appl Phys 1985;59(5):1428–33.

54. Javaheri S, Parker TJ, Wexler L, et al. Effect of theophylline on sleep-disordered breathing in heart failure. N Engl J Med 1996;335(8):562–7.

55. Andreas S, Reiter H, Luthje L, et al. Differential effects of theophylline on sympathetic excitation, hemodynamics, and breathing in congestive heart failure. Circulation 2004;110(15):2157–62.

56. Packer M, Carver JR, Rodeheffer RJ, et al. Effect of oral milrinone on mortality in severe chronic heart failure. The PROMISE study research group. N Engl J Med 1991;325(21):1468–75.

57. Javaheri S. Acetazolamide improves central sleep apnea in heart failure: a double-blind, prospective study. Am J Respir Crit Care Med 2006;173(2):234–7.

58. Wang TJ, Larson MG, Levy D, et al. Temporal relations of atrial fibrillation and congestive heart failure and their joint influence on mortality: the Framingham Heart Study. Circulation 2003;107(23):2920–5.

59. Rupprecht S, Hutschenreuther J, Brehm B, et al. Causality in the relationship between central sleep apnea and paroxysmal atrial fibrillation. Sleep Med 2008;9(4):462–4.

60. Leung RS, Huber MA, Rogge T, et al. Association between atrial fibrillation and central sleep apnea. Sleep 2005;28(12):1543–6.

61. Corra U, Pistono M, Mezzani A, et al. Sleep and exertional periodic breathing in chronic heart failure: prognostic importance and interdependence. Circulation 2006;113:44–50.

62. Brack T, Thuer I, Clarenbach CF, et al. Daytime Cheyne-Stokes respiration in ambulatory patients with severe congestive heart failure is associated with increased mortality. Chest 2007;132:1463–71.

63. Luo Q, Zhang HL, Tao XC, et al. Impact of untreated sleep apnea on prognosis of patients with congestive heart failure. Int J Cardiol 2010;144:420–2.

Central Sleep Apnea
The Complex Sleep Apnea Syndrome (CompSAS)

Bernardo J. Selim, MD[a], Mithri R. Junna, MD[b],
Timothy I. Morgenthaler, MD[a],*

KEYWORDS

- Central sleep apnea • Complex sleep apnea syndrome • Sleep-disordered breathing
- Obstructive sleep apnea syndrome • Treatment-emergent central sleep apnea
- Adaptive servoventilation

KEY POINTS

- Patients with complex sleep apnea syndrome (CompSAS) by definition first meet criteria for having obstructive sleep apnea syndrome, but on stabilization of the upper airway, demonstrate findings of central sleep apnea syndrome. Clinically, they resemble patients with obstructive sleep apnea syndrome, but may have underlying risk factors for central sleep apnea syndrome.
- Depending on the patient population being tested and the definition being used, CompSAS is present in between 3% and 20% of patients undergoing diagnostic polysomnography for suspected obstructive sleep apnea syndrome.
- Most patients with CompSAS will likely stabilize their ventilation with treatment focused on alleviating upper airway obstruction, such as continuous positive airway pressure, whereas some patients require noninvasive positive pressure ventilation. Adaptive servoventilation seems to be most reliable in improving ventilatory abnormalities.
- Studies so far have mostly evaluated different methods to reduce the apnea-hypopnea index rather than addressing patient-reported outcomes or downstream disease effects of CompSAS. Future studies should focus on patient-reported outcomes and downstream effects on disease or organ function, such as improvement in quality of life, sleep symptoms, cardiovascular endpoints, or mortality.

INTRODUCTION

Patients with sleep-disordered breathing (SDB) exhibit abnormal patterns of breathing most often characterized by inadequate maintenance of ventilation, in the form of either repetitive apneas or hypopneas, or as more sustained alveolar hypoventilation (which will not be discussed in this article). When most repetitive abnormal events are pathophysiologically related to upper airway obstruction during adequate efforts to breathe, obstructive sleep apnea syndrome (OSA) is diagnosed. In contrast, when most repetitive apneas and hypopneas result from transiently reduced efforts to breathe, central sleep apnea syndrome (CSA) is diagnosed. Complex sleep apnea syndrome (CompSAS) represents a combination of these 2 seemingly opposite ends of the spectrum of SDB phenotypes, obstructive and central sleep apnea.[1]

This description allows for considerable heterogeneity if not further refined, as there is a variety of

[a] Division of Pulmonary and Critical Care Medicine, Mayo Clinic Center for Sleep Medicine, Mayo Clinic, 200 First Street Southwest, Rochester, MN 55905, USA; [b] Department of Neurology, Mayo Clinic Center for Sleep Medicine, Mayo Clinic, 200 First Street Southwest, Rochester, MN 55905, USA
* Corresponding author.
E-mail address: tmorgenthaler@mayo.edu

Sleep Med Clin 9 (2014) 37–47
http://dx.doi.org/10.1016/j.jsmc.2013.10.004

ways to combine obstructive and central SDB. For example, one could find both types of SDB predominating at different times in the night, such as has been described in some patients with congestive heart failure, who manifest predominantly central sleep apnea initially, but more obstructive events later in the sleep period.[2] Alternatively, one might find central events predominating during non-rapid eye movement (NREM) sleep, but obstructive events during rapid eye movement (REM) sleep, or positional differences in the dominant type of SDB event.[3] Other permutations may be seen, but the most common descriptions in the literature are shown in **Table 1**. Using these definitions, CompSAS is reported in sleep laboratory populations from 3% to 20% of the time.

The most recently approved International Classification of Sleep Disorders, ICSD-II, does not provide a definition or diagnostic criteria for CompSAS. However, in a forthcoming update, it is proposed that CompSAS will be recognized as a form of central sleep apnea (possibly called "treatment-emergent central sleep apnea") and will be limited to the situation that arises when a patient has predominantly obstructive events during a diagnostic study (obstructive or mixed apneas, obstructive-appearing hypopneas) and has the persistence or emergence of central sleep apnea when obstructive events are resolved with positive airway pressure (PAP; without machine-provided breaths).[16] It is important to realize that by definition, all patients with CompSAS have OSA. It is proposed that any underlying cause for the revealed/emergent central sleep apnea, such as heart failure or opiate use, would exclude a diagnosis of CompSAS; instead, the patient would be diagnosed with both obstructive sleep apnea and the particular type of central sleep apnea. The intent of this refinement is to help segregate patients by cause wherever possible. Such refinement may help better delineate prevalence and clinical characteristics of patients with CompSAS. Time and further research will perhaps determine if this schema is merited as the pathophysiology of CompSAS becomes better understood.

EVALUATION
Clinical Characteristics

As stated above, CompSAS shares clinical features of both obstructive and central sleep apnea. OSA is characterized by increased upper airway resistance or obstruction accompanied by increased ventilatory effort, elevated critical closing pressure of the upper airway, and broadband low-frequency cardiopulmonary coupling.[17] In CSA, there is decreased ventilatory effort during disordered breathing events with variable critical closing pressure, and narrow-band low-frequency cardiopulmonary coupling. CompSAS shares physiologic properties of both, and central events often unmask when continuous positive airway pressure (CPAP) therapy or other therapies stabilize the upper airway (**Fig. 1**).

Patients with CompSAS represent a heterogeneous group, because there are several underlying processes that can lead to development of this condition. At baseline, their clinical characteristics are similar to those with OSA. They tend to be men, are obese with cardiovascular comorbidities, and complain of disrupted sleep or daytime sleepiness.[1,18] CompSAS is defined by demonstration of OSA during the diagnostic study followed by emergence of central sleep apnea during PAP therapy that tends to occur mostly frequently during NREM sleep.[18] The tendency to develop this unstable breathing pattern during PAP titration may be associated with additional cardiovascular comorbidity as well, including congestive heart failure and Cheyne-Stokes breathing pattern, arterial hypertension, and coronary artery disease.[6,12] However, up to one-third may have no identifiable risk factor.[19]

Polysomnographic Findings

Polysomnographically, the diagnostic study is characterized by predominantly obstructive events (obstructive or mixed apneas, obstructive hypopneas) with an apnea/hypopnea index (AHI) ≥ 5 per hour (**Fig. 2**). During PAP titration without a backup rate, significant resolution of obstructive events is demonstrated with the emergence or persistence of central apneas or hypopneas such that the central disordered breathing index is ≥ 5 per hour with greater than 50% central events (**Fig. 3**). In general, those with CompSAS may possess a mildly elevated central apnea index, particularly during NREM supine sleep, or higher arousal index during the diagnostic study when compared with those with pure OSA.[1,18,20] There has not been a notable difference in the presence or severity of periodic limb movements at baseline.[21] As outlined above, the central apnea index does increase with rising PAP therapy to control airway obstruction. Periodic limb movements have been noted to be less frequent on PAP therapy in those with CompSAS when compared with those with OSA.[21]

TREATMENT

In the most recent task force report on the treatment of adult CSA, CompSAS was not included in the guideline because this disorder is not part of the current ICSD-II nosology, and the evidence available was deemed "insufficient to establish treatment recommendations."[22] Controversies regarding treatment of CompSAS arise from the lack of consensus in the operational definition and a poor understanding of its pathophysiology. When diagnosing CompSAS, different authors have recruited heterogenous groups of subjects with not only obstructive sleep apnea physiology during the diagnostic polysomnographic study, but also with concomitant presence of central sleep apneas such as "mixed sleep apnea," Cheyne-Stokes respiration (CSR), or ataxic breathing. Even though most of these subjects may share common pathophysiologic pathways in the generation of central respiratory events, their primary trigger events could be as diverse as stroke, congestive heart failure, chronic opioid use, or high altitude. Therefore, the outcomes used to measure a successful response to treatment with CPAP devices and noninvasive ventilation conceivably could be tightly linked to the natural history of the triggering disease and its optimal treatment.

Several treatment modalities have been studied in patients with complex sleep apnea. CPAP, bilevel positive airway pressure without (BPAP-S) and with respiratory back up rate (BPAP-ST), and adaptive servo-ventilation (ASV) have been investigated. If those patients with baseline elevated apnea-hypopnea index but with low central apnea events (CAI<5/h) are focused on, in whom implementation of CPAP or BPAP shows emergence of central sleep apnea, the following conclusions can be drawn about treatment based on current evidence.

CPAP Therapy

Even though CPAP is the most successful and widely accepted treatment of obstructive sleep apnea, tolerance to CPAP treatment in patients with CSA tends to be lower.[23] By definition, patients with complex sleep apnea have emergent central sleep apneas while on PAP, a finding most often associated with increased total arousals, wake time after sleep onset, and sleep stages shift, making them a susceptible population for fragmented sleep and possible intolerance to CPAP therapy.[4] In a retrospective case control study comparing CPAP tolerance between obstructive sleep apnea and complex sleep apnea patients over 1 month, CompSAS patients showed greater difficulties to adapt to CPAP treatment based on need of earlier follow-ups for air hunger/dyspnea (8.8%, $P<.05$) and nocturnal unconscious mask removal (17.7%, $P<.05$), despite no

difference in CPAP pressure ($P = .112$) or subsequent compliance between groups (5.1 ± 1.6 vs 6.1 ± 1.5 h, $P = .156$).[4] In a large series of patients with CompSAS treated with CPAP for over 8 weeks, CPAP adherence was better when central apneas resolved than when it persisted.[9]

The degree of response and persistence of SDB while on CPAP therapy over time have been a controversial topic in sleep medicine. Some authors contend that most cases of CompSAS represent a transient phenomenon related to sleep fragmentation and sleep stage shifts that occur while on initial CPAP therapy,[9] the result of inadequate titration, or the overtitration of PAP resulting in Hering–Breuer reflex effect.[24] Indeed, Dernaika and colleagues[7] showed that after 2 to 3 months of CPAP treatment in CompSAS patients sufficient to eliminate obstructive events, 92% (14 of 21 patients) of patients have complete or near-complete resolution of CSA events by polysomnography. Javaheri and colleagues[9] found that in 33 of 44 patients who returned for follow-up CPAP titrations after 8 weeks of CPAP therapy, the central apneas had resolved. In both of these retrospective studies, more than one-third of patients treated with CPAP did not return for follow-up evaluation, so there is significant potential for bias. Another retrospective study by Kuzniar and colleagues[8] looked specifically at CompSAS patients returning for re-evaluation and found nearly 50% had persistent elevated central events despite compliance with CPAP therapy for a mean of 3 months. This study also likely has selection bias in that patients were having problems that eventuated in re-evaluation with polysomnography. Cassel and colleagues[12] have published the only prospective study reporting the impact of 3 months of fixed CPAP treatment in patients with CompSAS in comparison to those with only OSA. This study showed that the prevalence of CompSAS decreased from 12.2% at time of diagnosis to 6.9% (95% CI 4.5%–9.3%) while on CPAP treatment at 3 months. Those patients who continued to have CompSAS at follow-up were found to be older (61.0 vs 55.2 years; $P = .005$), have more coronary artery disease (40 vs 8.4%; $P = .001$), and have more fragmented sleep (46.5 vs 34.0; $P = .001$) than those without CompSAS.

Morgenthaler et al[25] have recently completed a prospective randomized multi-center trial comparing CPAP with ASV therapy for CompSAS over 90 days. Nearly 30% of those randomized to CPAP had persistent CompSAS at 90 days, while ASV was effective both acutely and over the 90 day period in controlling CompSAS in over 90% of patients. These data suggest that ASV will be more reliably effective therapy.

Table 1
Operational definition of CompSAS used by different authors in OSA patients while on CPAP titration trial

Author, Year	Operational Definition of CompSAS	Polysomnogram of CompSAS Patients (Median ± SD Events per Hour)	Comparison (No. of Patients)	Atrial Fibrillation at Baseline n (%)	Congestive Heart Failure at Baseline n (%)
Pusalavidyasagar et al,[4] 2006	Obstructive events (AHI <5), and emergent CAI ≥5 or CSR on CPAP	Diagnostic PSG: AHI 33.4/CAI 0.6 ± 1.3 CPAP trial PSG: AHI 24.6/CAI 19.4 ± 19	OSA (133) vs CompSAS (34) Follow-up 1 mo	CompSAS 4 (12)	CompSAS 3 (9)
Morgenthaler et al,[5] 2007	Obstructive events (AHI <5) and emergent CAI ≥5 or CSR on CPAP	Diagnostic PSG: AHI 49/ CAI 5.6 ± 4.6 CPAP trial PSG: AHI 41/ CAI 30.6 ± 18	ST-BiPAP vs ASV	CompSAS 1 (11.1)	CompSAS 1 (11.1)
Allam et al,[3] 2007	Obstructive events (AHI <5) and emergent CAI ≥5 or CSR on CPAP	Diagnostic PSG: AHI 49/ CAI 4.0 CPAP trial PSG: AHI 31/ CAI 15	Trial of CPAP, S-BiPAP, ST-BiPAP, and ASV in CompSAS (63) vs CSA (22) vs CSA/CSR (15)	CompSAS 16 (25)	CompSAS 16 (25)
Lehman et al,[6] 2007	Obstructive events (AHI <5) and emergence or persistence CAI ≥5 on CPAP	Diagnostic PSG: AHI 72/ CAI 12.4 ± 23 CPAP trial PSG: AHI 47.4/CAI 17 ± 14	OSA vs CompSAS	Not available	CompSAS 5 (38)
Dernaika et al,[7] 2007	Obstructive events (AHI <10) and emergent CAI ≥5 on CPAP	Diagnostic PSG: AHI 50.7/CAI 1.9 ± 2.1 CPAP trial PSG: AHI 14.9/CAI 11.1 ± 3.5	OSA (21) vs CompSAS (21) Follow-up 2–3 mo	None	None
Kuzniar et al,[8] 2008	Obstructive events (AHI <5) and emergent CAI ≥5 or CSR on CPAP	Diagnostic PSG: AHI 35/ CAI 0 CPAP trial PSG: AHI 20/ CAI 18 ± 9	CPAP responders (7) vs nonresponders (6) Follow-up 6 mo	Not available	Not available
Javaheri et al,[9] 2009	CPAP-emergent CSA: OSA, and residual CAI ≥5 on CPAP CPAP-persistent CSA: OSA, and persistent CAI ≥5 at baseline and during CPAP	Diagnostic PSG: AHI 57/ CAI 6 ± 11 CPAP trial PSG: AHI 27/ CAI 14 ± 20 (CPAP-CSA)	OSA (84) vs CPAP-emergent (6) and CPAP-persistent (27)	CPAP-CSA 7 (8.3)	CPAP-CSA 3 (3.6)

	Obstructive events definition	Diagnostic PSG	Comparison/Treatment		
Gilmartin et al,[10] 2010	Obstructive events (AHI <5) and emergent CAI ≥5 or persistent periodic breathing on CPAP	Diagnostic PSG: AHI 36/ CAI 3.8 ± 8.2 CPAP trial PSG: AHI 25/ CAI 8.9	CPAP + Enhanced expiratory rebreathing space (EERS)	CompSAS 20 (9.8)	CompSAS 22 (10.8)
Brown et al,[11] 2011	Obstructive events (AHI <5) and emergent or persistence CAI ≥5 on CPAP	Diagnostic PSG: AHI 36/ CAI 3.8 ± 8.2 CPAP trial PSG: AHI 25/ CAI 8.9	CPAP vs ASV	CompSAS 5 (20)	CompSAS 2 (8)
Cassel et al,[12] 2011	Obstructive events (AHI <5) and residual CAI ≥5 or periodic breathing on CPAP	Diagnostic PSG: AHI 35.9/CAI 2.0 CPAP trial PSG: AHI 10.4/CAI 7.4	OSA (593) vs CompSAS (82) Follow-up 3 mo	CompSAS 5 (6.1)	CompSAS 1 (1.2)
Bitter et al,[13] 2011	CAI ≥15 of central apnea or periodic breathing on CPAP and <10% of events being obstructive	Diagnostic PSG: AHI 30/ CAI not available CPAP trial PSG: CAI ≥15	CPAP vs ASV	CompSAS 8 (23)	CompSAS 34 (100)
Kuzniar et al,[14] 2011	Obstructive events (AHI <5) and emergent CAI ≥5 or CSR on CPAP	Diagnostic PSG: AHI 40–59/CAI 4–6 CPAP trial PSG: AHI 35–39/CAI 21–26	Comparison VPAP-AdaptSV vs BiPAP-AutoSV	Not available	CompSAS 5–8 (14–19)
Westhoff et al,[15] 2012	Obstructive events (AHI <5) and emergent CAI ≥5 on CPAP	Diagnostic PSG: AHI 40/ CAI 2 ± 2 CPAP trial PSG: AHI 34/ CAI 17 ± 8	Comparison Auto-CS2 vs BiPAP-AutoSV	CompSAS 5 (17)	Not available
Kuźniar et al,[1] 2012	Obstructive events (AHI <5) and emergent CAI ≥5 or CSR on CPAP	Diagnostic PSG: AHI 48/ CAI 0.5 CPAP trial PSG: AHI 32.5/CAI 21	CPAP vs S-BiPAP	N/A	CompSAS 10 (25.6)

Abbreviation: PSG, polysomnographic study.

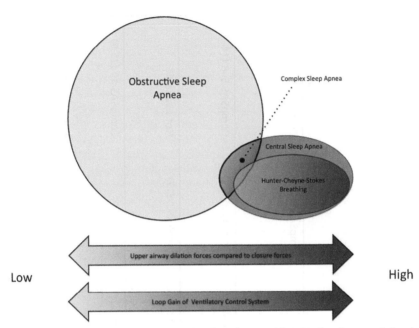

Fig. 1. CompSAS is a sleep-related breathing disorder that shares with OSA the characteristic of upper airway instability with propensity to collapse, and with central sleep apnea, including Hunter-Cheyne-Stokes breathing, the high loop gain of the ventilatory control system.

In conclusion, although most CompSAS patients tend to improve with long-term CPAP, there is a substantial group with persistently elevated CSA events who may likely benefit from therapies with greater emphasis on the elimination of the central respiratory events. Unfortunately, there are not well-defined clinical or polysomnographic criteria to preemptively identify the subgroup of CPAP nonresponders.

BPAP Therapy

Because of the uncertain response and poor tolerance of CSA to CPAP treatment, other treatment modalities such as BPAP-S and BPAP-ST have been tried. In a retrospective study published by Allam and colleagues,[3] they observed that patients with CompSAS on BPAP-S have a trend toward worsening of the AHI based on an increase in the number of central apneas in comparison to the same patients on CPAP treatment. This phenomenon could be explained by augmentation of ventilation during the hyperpneic phases of central sleep apnea breathing, thereby causing relative hypocapnia and increasing the risk of crossing the apneic threshold. Contrary to CPAP and BPAP-S, BPAP-ST has been shown to reduce total AHI by effectively eliminating central events, perhaps thereby reducing the tendency for hyperpnea in response to transient hypercapnia. Despite this reduction in AHI, total arousal index and respiratory arousal index were not

significantly different than the CPAP treatment group, showing a persistence of fragmented sleep.[3]

In summary, there is a paucity of publications regarding the impact of bilevel positive pressure ventilation in patient with CompSAS. The data available up to now discourage the use of BPAP-S mode in CompSAS. On the other hand, the BPAP-ST mode may offer a more effective alternative to CPAP in controlling respiratory events, even though the consolidation of sleep may still be suboptimal in certain patients.

ASV Therapy

The ASV is a feedback control system targeting minute ventilation ([ResMed Corp, San Diego, CA, USA] VPAP AdaptSV) or peak inspiratory flow ([Philips-Respironics, Andover, MA, USA], Bi-PAP AutoSV), adding a component of ventilation that is anticyclic to the patient's own respiratory drive periodicity.[19] Most of the experience with ASV is derived from the literature of CSR in the background of heart failure, but several studies have been published in CompSAS treatment.[23,26]

In comparison to CPAP and BPAP-ST, ASV treatment (ResMed, VPAP AdaptSV) in CompSAS patients has not only resulted in a significantly greater decrease of the AHI in all positions and stages of sleep, but also a lower residual arousal index, and a higher percentage of REM sleep (18% ASV vs 14% and 11%, respectively, for

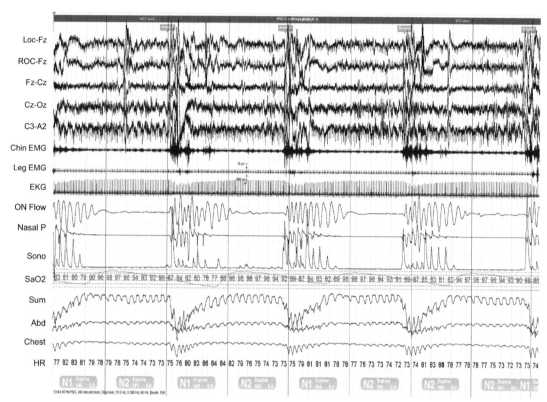

Fig. 2. Obstructive apneas-diagnostic portion of PSG. This polysomnographic segment obtained from a patient at clinical risk for obstructive sleep apnea shows 8 epochs of 30 seconds with cyclical obstructive apneic events. Each heavy vertical line demarks 30 seconds. The thermal sensor channel (ON flow) shows the presence of apneic events as a drop of ≥90% of peak thermal sensor signal from baseline. Most of these apneas are associated with arousals events (electroencephalogram, EEG) and clear oxyhemoglobin desaturations (see channel labeled SaO_2). Chin electromyogram (EMG) and leg EMG represent submental and pretibial EMGs. The electrocardiogram (EKG) shows sinus rhythm. Sono is a snoring microphone showing the opening of the collapsed upper airway with reinstitution of flow. Abdominal (Abd) and chest (Chest) respiratory impedance plethysmography signals demonstrate paradoxical breathing during apneic events. C3-A2, central EEG channel; Cz-Oz, occipital EEG channel; Fz-Cz, frontal EEG channel; HR, pulse rate (as read from the pulse oximeter); LOC-Fz, left electro-oculogram (EOG); ROC-Fz, right EOG.

BPAP-ST and CPAP; $P<.0001$).[3] Similar conclusions were drawn from a prospective randomized crossover clinical trial comparing BPAP-ST with ASV (ResMed, VPAP AdaptSV) in patients with CompSAS. Even though BPAP-ST was more effective in controlling AHI and respiratory arousal index in comparison to CPAP treatment (residual AHI 6.8 ± 6.8 vs 41.9 ± 28.1), the ASV was more effective than BPAP-ST in normalizing AHI (residual AHI 1.6 vs 6.8, $P = .02$) and respiratory arousal index in patients with CompSAS.[5] This beneficial effect should not be attributable to CompSAS patients with occult congestive heart failure. Westhoff and colleagues[15] showed that ASV was an effective therapy for CompSAS even in patients with normal brain natiuretic peptide, excluding possible confounding of CSA-CSR cases. In this population, ASV treatment led to a significant reduction in the AHI, from 40 ± 23 per hour while on CPAP to 4 ± 5 per hour after 6 weeks of ASV treatment. The arousal index and the Epworth Sleepiness Scale (ESS) score were also decreased during this period of treatment, from 36 ± 24 per hour to 20 ± 8 per hour, and the ESS decreased from 7.6 ± 4.9 to 4 ± 5 after 6 weeks of ASV.[15] In a study comparing success rates of ASV in treating patients with CompSAS in patients with congestive heart failure versus those with chronic opioid use, ASV was successful in reducing the AHI to less than 10 in 70.5% and 59.6%, respectively ($P = .236$).[27]

As mentioned above, 2 forms of servo ventilation are currently available in the United States, the VPAP-AdaptSV (ResMed) and the BIPAP-AutoSV (Respironics).[19] Both devices have comparative acute efficacy in control of AHI (median

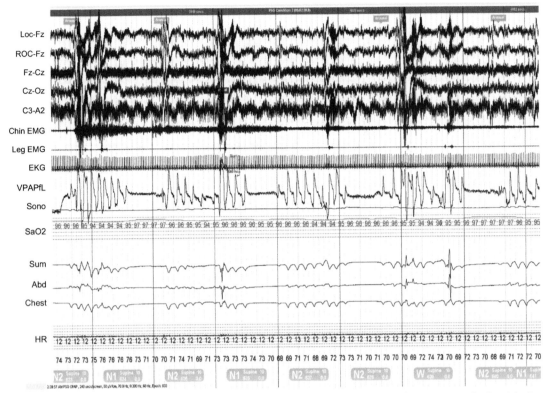

Fig. 3. CPAP emergent centrals – CPAP titration portion of PSG. This polysomnographic segment obtained during the CPAP titration shows 8 epochs of 30 seconds with cyclical central apneic events. Each heavy vertical line de-marks 30 seconds. The airflow signal from a continuous positive airway pressure unit, labeled (VPAPfL), shows the presence of cyclical apneic events. Most of these apneas are associated with arousals events (EEG) with relatively stable oxyhemoglobin saturations (see channel labeled SaO_2). Chin EMG and leg EMG represent submental and pretibial EMGs. The EKG shows sinus rhythm. Sono is a snoring microphone and is unremarkable. Abd and Chest respiratory impedance plethysmography signals demonstrate absence of respiratory efforts. C3-A2, central EEG channel; Cz-Oz, occipital EEG channel; Fz-Cz, frontal EEG channel; HR, pulse rate (as read from the pulse oxime-ter); LOC-Fz, left EOG; ROC-Fz, right EOG.

residual AHI 5 [interquartile range 2–11] in VPAP AdaptSV group and AHI 6 [3–13] in BIPAP-AutoSV group), with residual CAI not significantly different between treatment groups.[14] The compli-ance with both of them at 4 to 6 weeks was high, and the median Epworth Sleepiness Scale had improved by 2.5 (0–5) points in the VPAP AdaptSV group and 4 (1–9) points in the BIPAP-AutoSV group (P = .02).[14]

Another approach to stabilization of ventilation in CompSAS has been to use CPAP to splint the upper airway obstruction and use gasses, such as supplemental oxygen or low concentrations of carbon dioxide to reduce ventilatory instability.[10]

Adding dead space has also been shown effec-tive in some cases.[28] These treatments have not yet been tested in large series, and have not been widely used.

In conclusion, the ASV has emerged as a highly effective treatment option for patients with CompSAS, independent of the patient's clinical characteristics or response to other forms of nonin-vasive ventilation. Its use is associated not only with improvement of AHI, but also with sleep consolidation and improvement of daytime sleepi-ness (ESS) (**Fig. 4**). Both forms of servo ventilators available in United States, VPAP AdaptSV (ResMed Corp) and BiPAP AutoSV (Respironics), seem equally effective in the treatment of CompSAS and are associated with a generally high compliance.

OUTCOMES

There are no studies assessing long-term mortality or cardiovascular event outcomes in either treated or untreated CompSAS patients. However, if one regards CompSAS as either a form of OSA or CSA, one may draw some tentative conclusions. In the obstructive sleep apnea literature, it is well

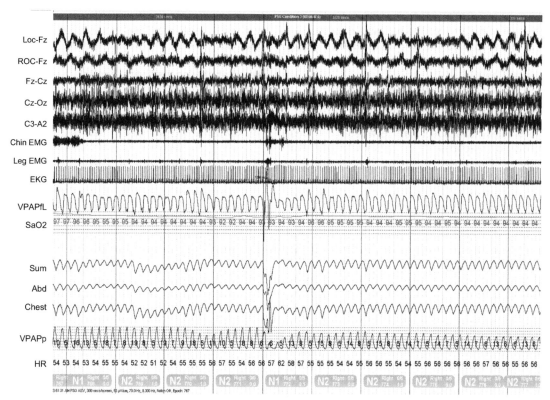

Fig. 4. Resolution of CPAP-emergent central apneas while on ASV treatment. This polysomnographic segment obtained during the ASV titration shows 8 epochs of 30 seconds with normalization of air flow. Each heavy vertical line demarks 30 seconds. The airflow signal from an ASV unit, labeled (VPAPfl) shows an end-expiratory pressure (EEP) of 5 cm H_2O and variable pressure support (PS). All central apneas are resolved. Stable oxyhemoglobin saturation is observed (see channel labeled SaO_2). Chin EMG and leg EMG represent submental and pretibial EMGs. The EKG shows sinus rhythm. Abd and Chest respiratory impedance plethysmography signals demonstrate normalization of respiratory efforts. C3-A2, central electroencephalogram (EEG) channel; Cz-Oz, occipital EEG channel; Fz-Cz, frontal EEG channel; HR, pulse rate (as read from the pulse oximeter); LOC-Fz, left EOG; ROC-Fz, right EOG.

documented that lack of appropriate treatment of severe disease (AHI ≥30 events per hour) is associated with increased morbidity and mortality in the short term (traffic and workplace accidents) and the long term (arterial hypertension and cardiovascular events).[29–32] PAP is the most cost-effective therapy for severe and symptomatic forms of OSA, and effective CPAP therapy has demonstrated a positive effect on blood pressure levels and the incidence of fatal and nonfatal cardiovascular events.[29,31,33–36] From the central sleep apnea literature, most of it derived from congestive heart failure patients with CSR; treatment with CPAP produces salutary outcomes only when it is effective in controlling the AHI. Effective treatment with ASV has shown improvement of cardiovascular outcomes such as clinical congestive heart failure stage, left ventricular ejection fraction, exercise tolerance, measures of chemoreceptor sensitivity, and serum N-terminal

pro-brain natriuretic peptide.[13] Even in cases of coexistence of OSA, CSA, and CSR in patients with and without heart failure, ASV reduced the central apnea hypopnea index and brain natiuretic peptide levels significantly more effectively as compared with CPAP over an 8-month and 12-month follow-up period.[37,38]

In summary, until additional data regarding short- and long-term outcomes of complex sleep apnea become available, the best treatment may well be the one that eliminates respiratory events, both obstructive and central in nature, leaving the patient with minimal residual excessive daytime sleepiness. At present there are no sound data to guide how long a CPAP trial should last before deciding that some more effective modality should be tried. The authors think that the decision must be based on the severity of residual abnormalities on initial introduction of CPAP, the likelihood of achieving close follow-up, and the symptoms and underlying cardiovascular risks the patient is carrying. The available data suggest that one should wait no longer than 8 to 12 weeks for reassessment if a conservative approach is decided on.

FOLLOW UP CARE

No studies have specifically evaluated the best follow-up practices. It is acknowledged that many of the problems encountered in adapting to PAP would be similar or even more significant in patients with CompSAS as compared with OSA or CSA. Extant literature indicates that adherence patterns are determined within the first days or weeks of therapy, so initial follow-up no later than 1 month is recommended, sooner if the patient is having problems adapting to therapy. At all follow-up visits, the patient should bring equipment and be able to relate to the sleep medicine practitioner successes and challenges encountered. Objective compliance and performance data may be downloaded from the device, and when combined with the clinical history, serve to guide the need for further evaluation or treatment changes. Once the patient is successful, and therapy is deemed effective, follow-up may be based on changes in the clinical situation (weight, heart function) and the need for periodic equipment checks. The authors tend to recommend annual follow-up for otherwise stable patients, although they are seeking ways to enhance the appropriateness of such follow-up visits.

SUMMARY

The CompSAS is now classified as a variant of CSA. Although it is not likely to be diagnosed before stabilizing the airway of patients with OSA during a diagnostic study, the physiologic substrate for CompSAS is present before initiation of CPAP, as evidenced by the ability to identify patients likely to develop CompSAS using analysis of cardiopulmonary coupling, and by its occurrence in patients whose OSA is treated using oral appliances. Treatment of CompSAS for now is aimed at correction of indices that indicate SDB, namely, normalization of the ventilatory pattern as evidenced by a reduced AHI and by smoothing of ventilatory effort. More meaningful outcomes of therapy, such as improved alertness, cognition, and cardiovascular outcomes, await further large prospective randomized controlled trials, but for now, it seems reasonable to apply principles similar to those applied when assessing adequacy of outcomes for OSA and CSA. For most patients, this will likely mean a trial of CPAP to stabilize

the upper airway, and then in those who do not normalize their breathing pattern, or who are deemed unlikely to normalize their breathing pattern, treatment with ASV, or other therapies aimed at altering ventilatory control.

REFERENCES

1. Kuźniar TJ, Morgenthaler TI. Treatment of complex sleep apnea syndrome. Chest 2012;142:1049–57.
2. Tkacova R, Niroumand M, Lorenzi-Filho G, et al. Overnight shift from obstructive to central apneas in patients with heart failure: role of PCO2 and circulatory delay. Circulation 2001;103:238–43.
3. Allam JS, Olson EJ, Gay PC, et al. Efficacy of adaptive servoventilation in treatment of complex and central sleep apnea syndromes. Chest 2007;132:1839–46.
4. Pusalavidyasagar SS, Olson EJ, Gay PC, et al. Treatment of complex sleep apnea syndrome: a retrospective comparative review. Sleep Med 2006;7:474–9.
5. Morgenthaler TI, Gay PC, Gordon N, et al. Adaptive servoventilation versus noninvasive positive pressure ventilation for central, mixed, and complex sleep apnea syndromes. Sleep 2007;30:468–75.
6. Lehman S, Antic NA, Thompson C, et al. Central sleep apnea on commencement of continuous positive airway pressure in patients with a primary diagnosis of obstructive sleep apnea-hypopnea. J Clin Sleep Med 2007;3:462–6.
7. Dernaika T, Tawk M, Nazir S, et al. The significance and outcome of continuous positive airway pressure-related central sleep apnea during split-night sleep studies. Chest 2007;132:81–7.
8. Kuzniar TJ, Pusalavidyasagar S, Gay PC, et al. Natural course of complex sleep apnea–a retrospective study. Sleep Breath 2008;12:135–9.
9. Javaheri S, Smith J, Chung E. The prevalence and natural history of complex sleep apnea. J Clin Sleep Med 2009;5:205–11.
10. Gilmartin G, McGeehan B, Vigneault K, et al. Treatment of positive airway pressure treatment-associated respiratory instability with enhanced expiratory rebreathing space (EERS). J Clin Sleep Med 2010;6:529–38.
11. Brown SE, Mosko SS, Davis JA, et al. A retrospective case series of adaptive servoventilation for complex sleep apnea. J Clin Sleep Med 2011;7:187–95.
12. Cassel W, Canisius S, Becker HF, et al. A prospective polysomnographic study on the evolution of complex sleep apnoea. Eur Respir J 2011;38:329–37.
13. Bitter T, Westerheide N, Hossain MS, et al. Complex sleep apnoea in congestive heart failure. Thorax 2011;66:402–7.

14. Kuzniar TJ, Patel S, Nierodzik CL, et al. Comparison of two servo ventilator devices in the treatment of complex sleep apnea. Sleep Med 2011; 12:538–41.

15. Westhoff M, Arzt M, Litterst P. Prevalence and treatment of central sleep apnoea emerging after initiation of continuous positive airway pressure in patients with obstructive sleep apnoea without evidence of heart failure. Sleep Breath 2012;16:71–8.

16. Berry R. Challenges in the diagnosis of sleep related breathing disorders, in Workshop at Sleep 2013: case studies in the application of the ICSD III. Baltimore, June 4, 2013.

17. Thomas RJ, Mietus JE, Peng CK, et al. Differentiating obstructive from central and complex sleep apnea using an automated electrocardiogram-based method. Sleep 2007;30:1756–69.

18. Morgenthaler TI, Kagramanov V, Hanak V, et al. Complex sleep apnea syndrome: is it a unique clinical syndrome? Sleep 2006;29:1203–9.

19. Kuzniar TJ, Morgenthaler TI. Adaptive servoventilation in treatment of sleep-disordered breathing. In: Clete K, editor. Encyclopedia of sleep. Waltham (MA): Academic Press; 2013. p. 510–9.

20. Yaegashi H, Fujimoto K, Abe H, et al. Characteristics of Japanese patients with complex sleep apnea syndrome: a retrospective comparison with obstructive sleep apnea syndrome. Intern Med 2009;48:427–32.

21. Pusalavidyasagar S, Kuzniar TJ, Olson EJ, et al. Periodic limb movements in complex sleep apnea syndrome. Open Sleep J 2009;2:43–7.

22. Aurora RN, Chowdhuri S, Ramar K, et al. The treatment of central sleep apnea syndromes in adults: practice parameters with an evidence-based literature review and meta-analyses. Sleep 2012;35:17–40.

23. Philippe C, Stoïca-Herman M, Drouot X, et al. Compliance with and effectiveness of adaptive servoventilation versus continuous positive airway pressure in the treatment of Cheyne-Stokes respiration in heart failure over a six month period. Heart 2006;92: 337–42.

24. Malhotra A, Bertisch S, Wellman A. Complex sleep apnea: it isn't really a disease. J Clin Sleep Med 2008;4:406–8.

25. Morgenthaler TI, Kuzniar TJ, Wolfe LF, et al, The Complex Sleep Apnea Resolution Study: A Prospective Randomized Controlled Trial of Continuous Positive Airway Pressure vs. Adaptive Servoventilation Therapy. Accepted in Sleep, 2014.

26. Teschler H, Döhring J, Wang Y, et al. Adaptive pressure support servo-ventilation. A novel treatment for Cheyne-Stokes respiration in heart failure. Am J Respir Crit Care Med 2001;164:614–9.

27. Ramar K, Ramar P, Morgenthaler TI. Adaptive servo-ventilation in patients with central or complex sleep apnea related to chronic opioid use and congestive heart failure. J Clin Sleep Med 2012;8:569–76.

28. Thomas RJ. Effect of added dead space to positive airway pressure for treatment of complex sleep-disordered breathing. Sleep Med 2005;6(2):177–8.

29. Barbe, Pericas J, Munoz A, et al. Automobile accidents in patients with sleep apnea syndrome. An epidemiological and mechanistic study. Am J Respir Crit Care Med 1998;158:18–22.

30. Teran-Santos J, Jimenez-Gomez A, Cordero-Guevara J. The association between sleep apnea and the risk of traffic accidents. Cooperative Group Burgos-Santander. N Engl J Med 1999;340:847–51.

31. Marin JM, Carrizo SJ, Vicente E, et al. Long-term cardiovascular outcomes in men with obstructive sleep apnoea-hypopnoea with or without treatment with continuous positive airway pressure: an observational study. Lancet 2005;365:1046–53.

32. Peppard PE, Young T, Palta M, et al. Prospective study of the association between sleep-disordered breathing and hypertension. N Engl J Med 2000; 342:1378–84.

33. Sanders MH, Montserrat JM, Farre R, et al. Positive pressure therapy: a perspective on evidence-based outcomes and methods of application. Proc Am Thorac Soc 2008;5:161–72.

34. Duran-Cantolla J, Aizpuru F, Montserrat JM, et al. Continuous positive airway pressure as treatment for systemic hypertension in people with obstructive sleep apnoea: randomised controlled trial. BMJ 2010;341:c5991.

35. Barbe F, Duran-Cantolla J, Capote F, et al. Long-term effect of continuous positive airway pressure in hypertensive patients with sleep apnea. Am J Respir Crit Care Med 2010;181:718–26.

36. Martinez-Garcia MA, Campos-Rodriguez F, Catalan-Serra P, et al. Cardiovascular mortality in obstructive sleep apnea in the elderly: role of long-term continuous positive airway pressure treatment: a prospective observational study. Am J Respir Crit Care Med 2012;186:909–16.

37. Randerath WJ, Nothofer G, Priegnitz C, et al. Long-term auto-servoventilation or constant positive pressure in heart failure and coexisting central with obstructive sleep apnea. Chest 2012;142:440–7.

38. Randerath WJ, Galetke W, Stieglitz S, et al. Adaptive servo-ventilation in patients with coexisting obstructive sleep apnoea/hypopnoea and Cheyne-Stokes respiration. Sleep Med 2008;9:823–30.

Opioid-Induced Central Sleep Apnea: Mechanisms and Therapies

Shahrokh Javaheri, MD[a,b,*], Winfried J. Randerath, MD[c]

KEYWORDS

- Opioids • Methadone • Buprenorphine • Central sleep apnea • Complex sleep apnea
- Adaptive servoventilation

KEY POINTS

- Chronic opioid use is an established risk factor for central sleep apnea (CSA), as shown by a high prevalence of CSA in this population. CSA is eliminated with withdrawal of opioids, and animal experimentations have shown potential mechanisms.
- CSA may be present on initial diagnostic polysomnography or it may emerge with initiation of continuous positive airway pressure therapy, referred to as complex sleep apnea.
- The first approach to therapy is programmed withdrawal of opioids, if possible.
- For patients with complex sleep apnea and those patients whose diagnostic polysomnographies show CSA, we have used servoventilators effectively.
- Long-term randomized clinical trials are needed to determine if effective treatment of CSA improves quality of life and the excess mortality of patients using opioids.

INTRODUCTION

While asleep, patients using chronic opioids are at risk for developing a variety of disordered breathing events[1] which are unmasked by the profound effect of the state of sleep on breathing. These sleep-related breathing disorders (SRBDs) are complex and include unique patterns of irregular breathing, with both obstructive and central apneas and hypopneas, and hypoventilation characterized by sustained hypoxemia and hypercapnia. Many opioid users are found dead in bed and at autopsy no cause is found. It is well known that the sine qua non of opioid intoxication is a terminal lethal apnea. It is speculated that the spectrum of opioid-induced sleep-disordered breathing is also the cause of increased mortality in chronic users of opioids. In addition, some individuals have died postoperatively in part related to administration of opioids. The fatality has been particularly noticeable after tonsillectomy with administration of codeine for pain.[2] For a variety of reasons, but particularly in patients with psychiatric disorders, many patients on opioids are also on benzodiazepines. This combination may be particularly fatal, because these 2 classes of drugs are agonists for 2 different receptors with adverse effects on breathing, the former on the μ receptor and the latter on the γ-aminobutyric acid receptor.

In recent years, use of opioid medications has increased dramatically. The commonest indications of opioids include chronic pain syndromes, relief of postoperative pain, therapy for opioid dependency, and, at times, relief of dyspnea associated with chronic obstructive pulmonary disease. Between 1997 and 2007, prescriptions for opioid analgesics increased by 700%. During the same period, the number of grams of prescribed methadone increased by more than 1200%.[3] The reason for escalation in opioid prescriptions since 1997 is

[a] University of Cincinnati College of Medicine, Cincinnati, OH, USA; [b] Sleepcare Diagnostics, 4780 Socialville Fosters Road, Mason, OH 45040, USA; [c] Institute of Pneumology at the University Witten/Herdecke, Clinic for Pneumology and Allergology, Center of Sleep Medicine and Respiratory Care, Solingen, Germany
* Corresponding author. Sleepcare Diagnostics, 4780 Socialville Fosters Road, Mason, OH 45040.
E-mail address: javaheri@snorenomore.com

Sleep Med Clin 9 (2014) 49–56
http://dx.doi.org/10.1016/j.jsmc.2013.10.003
1556-407X/14/$ – see front matter © 2014 Elsevier Inc. All rights reserved.

multifactorial and includes increased awareness by health care providers of treating chronic pain and awareness of patients of seeking treatment. Furthermore, in 1997, a joint statement by the American Pain Society and the American Academy of Pain Medicine[4] implied that it is acceptable to use opioids for the treatment of chronic pain with minimal risk of respiratory depression. We suspect that this position was based on the observation that chronic respiratory acidosis, a reflection of long-term respiratory depression, is not common or is mild in most cases. However, at that time, sleep studies were not performed in patients using opioids. It is now clear that while individuals are asleep, opioid-induced respiratory depression is unmasked and SRBDs become highly prevalent in patients using opioids. Another similar misconception relates to the acceleration in the use of semisynthetic buprenorphine for therapy for opioid dependency. The retail distribution of buprenorphine increased 7000-fold from 107 g in 2002 to more than 800,000 g in 2008.[5] Being an opioid partial μ-agonist, buprenorphine has been perceived to have a better safety profile in regards to respiratory depression when compared with other full μ-agonists such as methadone. However, as discussed later, buprenorphine is a potential cause of severe SRBDs as well.[5]

SRBDs, both obstructive and central events, are highly prevalent in patients on opioids.[1,5–13] However, the focus of this review is opioid-induced central sleep apnea (CSA), which is observed in 2 specific circumstances. CSA may be found during initial polysomnographic study or it may emerge with continuous positive airway pressure (CPAP) therapy in individuals whose initial polysomnography showed obstructive sleep apnea (OSA).[14,15] The latter is referred to as complex sleep apnea. These 2 kinds of CSA are discussed later.

CSA Present During Initial Polysomnographic Study

These patients may present with symptoms suggestive of OSA, with a history of habitual snoring and daytime sleepiness.[15] Commonly, such patients are not obese. Polysomnography shows presence of either CSA as the predominant form of sleep apnea, or CSA mixed with both OSAs and hypopneas (**Fig. 1**). As discussed later, the importance of this polysomnographic finding is that the CSA remains CPAP resistant, and such patients invariably require treatment with adaptive servoventilation.

Several large observational studies of patients receiving full (not partial) opioids agonists have shown high prevalence of CSA, defined as a central apnea index (CAI) of 5 or more per hour of sleep. In the aforementioned studies, patients were treated with full opioid agonists. In a recent study, Farney and colleagues[5] performed

5 min epoch

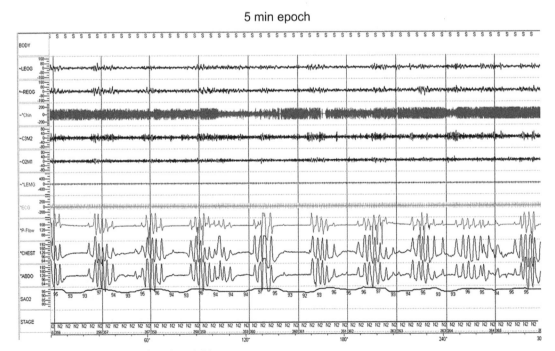

Fig. 1. CSA in a patient on chronic opioids.

polysomnography in 70 consecutive patients who were admitted for therapy with buprenorphine. Buprenorphine is a semisynthetic opioid with partial μ-agonist activity and has been widely used for therapy for opioid dependency since 1969. Being a partial agonist, it was believed to have minimal respiratory suppression when compared with full agonists. For this reason, many patients have been treated with this drug. In this important study,[5] 61% had an apnea-hypopnea index (AHI) of 5 or more per hour of sleep, 33% had moderate sleep apnea with an AHI of 15 to less than 30 per hour of sleep and 17% had severe sleep apnea defied by an AHI of 30 or more per hour of sleep. The mean AHI was 20 per hour, of which CAI was 11 per hour. The mean obstructive apnea index was 2 per hour. This study shows that buprenorphine has respiratory depressant properties, as do other opioids.

Combining the results of 5 studies of relatively large numbers of patients using opioids (**Table 1**),[5,8,11–13] 35% had CAI of 5 or more per hour of sleep. However, 20% and 10% of patients had, respectively, CAI of 15 or higher and 30 or higher per hour of sleep. These SRBDs are frequently associated with arousals, and with desaturation, particularly in patients with low baseline arterial oxyhemoglobin saturation, not uncommon findings in patients on opioids.

The pattern of breathing and central apneas caused by chronic opioid use has unique characteristics (see **Fig. 1**). This recognizable polysomnographic pattern is completely different from another recognizable pattern referred to as Hunter-Cheyne-Stokes breathing, observed in patients with congestive heart failure. Hunter-Cheyne-Stokes breathing is a form of periodic breathing characterized by crescendo and decrescendo changes in airflow or tidal volume, with a central apnea in the midst (**Fig. 2**).[16] In contradistinction, opioid-induced CSA occurs amid 2 respiratory patterns, which are observed in the same patient (**Fig. 1**). First, Biot ataxic breathing, described by Camille Biot in 1897 in a patient with tuberculous meningitis,[17] is common in patients on opioids. This irregular breathing pattern is characterized by variability in breathing rate, amplitude of tidal volume, and duration of central apneas. The second pattern is cluster breathing and is characterized by cycles of deep breaths, in which the amplitude of tidal volume is relatively stable, with interspersed central apneas of variable duration. In our experience with opioid-induced CSA, cluster breathing is more commonly observed than ataxic breathing.

As noted earlier, there is a distinct difference between the patterns of breathing in heart failure versus opioids. Another distinct difference is the duration of central apneas, which are variable with opioids, but not in heart failure. However, 1 similarity is emphasized: both in congestive heart failure and in opioids, central apneas primarily occurred in non–rapid eye movement (NREM) sleep. This situation has to do with neurophysiology of rapid eye movement sleep, which is not conducive to pathophysiologic mechanisms of central apnea.[18]

Opioid-Associated Complex Sleep Apnea

In this condition, the patient using an opioid presents with symptoms consistent with OSA, such as habitual snoring and excessive daytime sleepiness, although obesity may not be present.[15] Diagnostic polysomnography shows OSA without or with occasional central apneas. However, many central apneas emerge during initiation of CPAP therapy, with CAI of at least 5 per hour of sleep. AHI remains abnormally increased. This situation has been referred to as complex sleep apnea. There is frequently persistence of central apneas with commencement of CPAP therapy in patients whose initial diagnostic polysomnography also shows presence of central apneas. Distinction should be made between these 2 conditions.

Guilleminault and colleagues[14] have reported on the prevalence of complex sleep apnea in patients taking opioids. These patients underwent polysomnography, which showed severe OSA with an average AHI of 44/h. The mean CAI was less than 1/h of sleep. However, with CPAP treatment, CSA emerged and mean CAI increased to 14/h of sleep. As discussed later, central apneas were eliminated with the use of bilevel devices with backup rate.

Table 1
Prevalence of CSA (CAI ≥5) in 5 large studies

	n	n ≥5	n ≥15	n ≥30
Mogri et al,[12] 2009	98	43	NR	NR
Webster et al,[11] 2008	147	48	34	21
Wang et al,[8] 2005	50	17	NR	1
Sharkey et al,[13] 2010	71	23	10	NR
Farley et al,[9]	70	21	14	6
Total	436	152/436 35%	58/288 20%	28/267 10%

Abbreviation: NR, not reported.

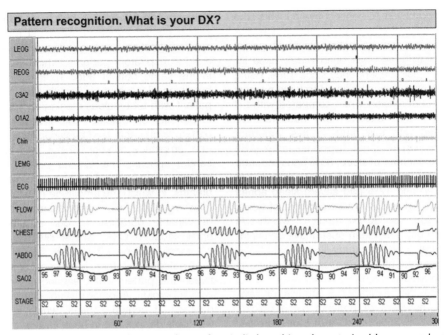

Pattern recognition. What is your DX?

Fig. 2. Hunter-Cheyne-Stokes breathing is a form of periodic breathing characterized by crescendo and decrescendo changes in airflow or tidal volume, with a central apnea in the midst. This patient is 80 years old, with history of chronic heart failure and reduced ejection fraction.

MECHANISMS OF OPIOID-INDUCED CSA

Two mechanisms that could mediate opioid-induced CSA are discussed: the first is suppression of breathing rhythm, and the second, alterations in ventilatory control.

Suppression of Breathing Rhythm

Results of 2 sets of animal studies from different laboratories, one in neonatal rats and the other in adult rodents, are consistent with this notion. From experiments in neonatal rat brain stem, Feldman and colleagues[19,20] concluded that the pre-Botzinger complex (pre-BotC) located in the ventrolateral medullary portion of the brain stem is the dominant site for inspiration. The pre-BotC contains μ opioid receptors, and stimulation with μ opioid agonists suppresses the rate of breathing. In anesthetized adult rats,[21] continuous local unilateral application of the μ opioid receptor agonists ([D- Ala 2, N-Me Phe 4, Gly-ol]-enkephalin) DAMGO or fentanyl into the pre-BotC caused prolongation in expiratory time and slowing of respiratory rate. At higher doses of agonists, complete cessation of diaphragmatic muscle activity (ie, central apnea) occurred. These changes were reversed by the μ opioid receptor antagonist naloxone. These alterations in breathing pattern were also observed in naturally sleeping rats in NREM sleep. Therefore, these animal studies

indicate that opioids cause a state-dependent respiratory rate depression, which is most profound in NREM sleep and during anesthesia. The latter finding has important implications in regards to anesthesia in humans in whom, as noted earlier, opioids are used to suppress postoperative pain, with consequent risk of mortality.

Alterations in ventilatory control

The second potential mechanism that could result in CSA is a combination of increased controller and plant gains.[18] The controller gain is defined by the sensitivity of the peripheral arterial and central chemoreceptors to hypoxia and hypercapnia (the slope of the hypoxic and hypercapnic ventilatory responses, respectively). The higher the controller gain, the higher the likelihood of developing CSA. In 1 study,[22] patients on chronic opioids showed increased hypoxic ventilatory response (increased controller gain) during wakefulness. Increased hypoxic ventilatory response during sleep could increase the likelihood of developing central apnea. However, in contrast, opioids have been shown to decrease the sensitivity to CO_2,[22] which could negate increased hypoxic chemosensitivity.

Plant gain is defined as the change in arterial Pco_2 (partial pressure of carbon dioxide) for a given change in ventilation. Furthermore, opioids may also cause chronic hypercapnia, which increases plant gain.[18] This aspect of ventilatory control altered by opioids has been discussed in detail elsewhere[1] and is briefly reviewed.

However, as noted, opioids have been shown to decrease the sensitivity to CO_2,[22] which could negate hypoxic chemosensitivity.

Plant gain is defined as the change in arterial P_{CO_2} for a given change in ventilation. Opioids may decrease alveolar ventilation, resulting in hypercapnia (increased plant gain). In that case, as dictated by the metabolic hyperbola defining the relationship of alveolar ventilation with arterial P_{CO_2} (for a given metabolic rate), a small increase in ventilation decreases P_{CO_2} considerably. If this decrease occurs while the patient is asleep, and P_{CO_2} decreases lower than the apneic threshold, central apneas occur.[18]

It is conceivable that a combination of increased hypoxic ventilatory response and increased plant gain collectively increase the loop gain and result in central apneas during sleep.

TREATMENT OPTIONS FOR OPIOID-INDUCED CSA

There are several potential options for treatment of opioid-induced CSA.[1] However, except for withdrawal from opioids, a difficult task, and the use of adaptive servoventilation and bilevel pressure devices in S/T mode (**Fig. 3**), no other alternative has been systematically studied. When possible, supervised withdrawal of opioids should eliminate CSA, but this is difficult to achieve. In case reports, successful withdrawal of opioids resolved sleep-disordered breathing in addition to improving daytime sleepiness.[23,24]

Our studies have shown that administration of acetazolamide, theophylline, or supplemental oxygen improves CSA in heart failure.[25] It is important to determine if these drugs improve CSA induced by opioids. In a case report of a patient on a long-acting opioid who had OSA and who developed complex sleep apnea on CPAP, CSA was eliminated by addition of single-dose acetazolamide, 250 mg, before bedtime.[26] In a double-blind, randomized clinical trial,[27] we previously reported that 250 mg acetazolamide administered 30 minutes before bedtime was effective in the treatment of CSA in heart failure. A similarly designed study of opioid-induced CSA is needed.

Another group of drugs that could be effective is the ampakines, a family of compounds that modulate amino-3-hydroxy-5-methyl-4-isoxazole-propionate (AMPA) receptors. This is the receptor for the excitatory neurotransmitter, glutamate, and glutamate-mediated neurotransmission at the AMPA receptors in pre-BotC has excitatory inspiratory drive. Using rat models, Greer and Ren[28] and Ren and colleagues[29] showed that the ampakines alleviate opiate-induced respiratory depression of central respiratory rhythmogenesis. In a study of 16 healthy human individuals,[30] CX717 counteracted alfentanil-induced respiratory depression without affecting opiate-mediated analgesia. Human studies are needed to determine if the ampakines reverse opioid-induced central apneas during sleep. Unless studies are performed to show efficacy, routine use of ampakines is not recommended. Our current recommendations to treat sleep apnea comorbid with use of opioids are titration with positive airway pressure devices (PAP), depending on the polysomnographic findings (see **Fig. 3**), as described later.

Treatment of OSA with PAP Devices in Patients on Opioids

CPAP devices have been successfully used for treatment of OSA in the general population. We also recommend CPAP to treat OSA in patients

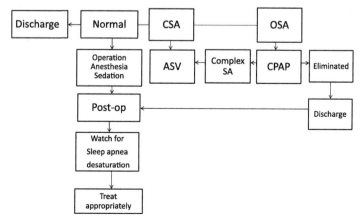

Fig. 3. Patients on chronic opioids and also before any surgery should undergo polysomnography.

on opioids, because we have had great success. However, in some patients whose polysomnographies show OSA, therapy with CPAP fails and CSA emerges, a condition referred to as complex sleep apnea. Complex sleep apnea is also observed when patients with OSA, particularly those with severe OSA, and without opioid exposure, are treated with CPAP.[31] There are no systematic studies to determine if prevalence of complex sleep apnea is higher in groups of patients with exposure to opioids compared with those not exposed to opioids. However, Guilleminault and colleagues[14] reported a high prevalence of complex sleep apnea in 44 patients with severe OSA on chronic opioid therapy. In these patients, either bilevel devices with backup rate or an adaptive servoventilation (ASV) device should be effective, as discussed later.

Treatment of CSA with PAP Devices in Patients on Opioids

CPAP has been used to effectively treat CSA associated with congestive heart failure. However, in almost 50% of these patients, CSA is not suppressed by CPAP.[32,33] In patients with heart failure in whom CSA is not suppressed by CPAP, continued use of CPAP is associated with excess mortality,[33] and we have recommended[34] that CPAP should not be used if after the night of titration, CSA is not suppressed. In these patients, we recommend ASV titration, and observational studies show improved survival in these patients with heart failure.[35,36]

In contrast to heart failure, application of CPAP to treat CSA associated with opioids has proved ineffective,[15,37,38] and treatment with an ASV device is recommended to begin with (ie, without a trial of CPAP). In a large retrospective study, Allam and colleagues[38] observed many failures with initiation of CPAP therapy in patients on opioid-induced CSA. These patients were successfully treated with an ASV device. We reported[15] 5 patients with severe central and OSA (AHI = 70, CAI = 26) who failed CPAP therapy despite continued use of CPAP for several weeks. Our further experience (unpublished data) with these patients has been confirmatory, and we have concluded that continued use of CPAP fails and therefore have abandoned recommending CPAP therapy for opioid-induced CSA (this is in contrast to patients with heart failure).

Therefore, for all opioid patients whose diagnostic polysomnogram shows CSA, the recommended positive airway pressure devices are either ASV[15,38] or bilevel devices in S/T mode.[39] This is also the case for patients on opioids with

complex sleep apnea, in whom CSA emerges during CPAP therapy. As noted earlier, Guilleminault and colleagues studied 44 chronic opioid users with OSA (mean AHI = 44) who developed complex sleep apnea with commencement of CPAP titration (CAI increased from .06 on the diagnostic polysomnography to 14/h with CPAP). CSA persisted with bilevel therapy as well (CAI = 12/h). However, bilevel with backup rate was effective (CAI = 2/h).

Although the operation of bilevel devices is well known, the algorithms of the pressure support servoventilators (VPAP Adapt (ResMed Corp, San Deigo, CA) and BiPAP Auto SV Advanced System 1 (Phillips Respironics, Murrysville, PA) and SomnoVent CR (Weinmann Medical Technology, Hamburg, Germany; not available in United States) are complex and not well known among sleep physicians and technologists. The description of algorithms of ASV devices can be found elsewhere[40–43] and is beyond the scope of this review. However, the 3 devices have common features, including algorithms for backup rate in order to abort the time course of central apneas. The newest generation of ASV devices are equipped with automatic algorithms for end-expiratory positive airway pressure control, like auto-CPAP to eliminate obstructive disordered breathing events. The third common feature of ASV devices relates to algorithms for automatic variable anticyclic pressure support. The positive inspiratory pressure is modulated in such a way to counterbalance the patient's current level of ventilation. With this platform, dynamic anticyclic pressure support is applied during the undershoot period of ventilation and a deaugmentation occurs during the overshoot of ventilation. Therefore, ASV devices are particularly effective in patients with hybrid SRBD, such as found in patients on opioids.[44]

Three studies from 2 centers have shown effectiveness of an ASV device.[15,38,45] However, appropriate titration is critical to a successful result,[15,46] otherwise failure may occur.

SUMMARY

Chronic opioid use is an established risk factor for CSA, as shown by a high prevalence of CSA in this population. CSA is eliminated with withdrawal of opioids, and animal experimentations have shown potential mechanisms. CSA may be present on initial diagnostic polysomnography or it may emerge with initiation of CPAP therapy, referred to as complex sleep apnea. The first approach to therapy is programmed withdrawal of opioids, if possible. This is a difficult task. CPAP therapy is recommended for those with OSA, and development of complex sleep apnea should be looked for. For the latter patients and those patients whose diagnostic polysomnographies show CSA, we have used servoventilators effectively. Bilevel devices in the S/T mode are another alternative. However, long-term randomized clinical trials are needed to determine if effective treatment of CSA improves quality of life and the excess mortality of patients using opioids.

REFERENCES

1. Cao M, Javaheri S. Chronic opioid use: effects on respiration and sleep. In: Tvildiani D, Gegechkori K, editors. Opioids pharmacology, clinical uses and adverse effects. New York: NovaScience; 2012. p. 1–13.

2. Kelly LE, Riedr M, van den Anker J, et al. More codeine fatalities after tonsillectomy in North American children. Pediatrics 2012;129:e1343–7.

3. Boyer EW. Management of opioid analgesic overdose. N Engl J Med 2012;167:146–55.

4. American Academy of Pain Medicine and American Pain Society. The use of opioid for chronic pain. Clin J Pain 1997;13:6–8.

5. Farney RJ, Mc Donald AM, Boyle KM, et al. Sleep-disordered breathing in patients receiving therapy with buprenorphine /naloxone. Eur Respir J 2013; 42(2):394–403.

6. Randerath WJ, George S. Opioid-induced sleep apnea: is it a real problem. J Clin Sleep Med 2012;8: 577–8.

7. Teichtahl H, Prodromidis A, Miller B, et al. Sleep-disordered breathing in stable methadone programme patients: a pilot study. Addiction 2001;96: 395–403.

8. Wang D, Teichtahl H, Drummer O, et al. Central sleep apnea in stable methadone maintenance treatment patients. Chest 2005;128:1348–56.

9. Farney RJ, Walker JM, Cloward TV, et al. Sleep-disordered breathing associated with long-term opioid therapy. Chest 2003;123:632–9.

10. Walker JM, Farney RJ, Rhondeau SM, et al. Chronic opioid use is a risk factor for the development of central sleep apnea and ataxic breathing. J Clin Sleep Med 2007;3:455–61.

11. Webster LR, Choi Y, Desai H, et al. Sleep-disordered breathing and chronic opioid therapy. Pain Med 2008;9:425–32.

12. Mogri M, Desai H, Webster L, et al. Hypoxemia in patients on chronic opiate therapy with and without sleep apnea. Sleep Breath 2009;13:49–57.

13. Sharkey KM, Kurth ME, Anderson BJ, et al. Obstructive sleep apnea is more common than central sleep apnea in methadone maintenance patients with subjective sleep complaints. Drug Alcohol Depend 2010;108:77–83.

14. Guilleminault C, Cao M, Yue HJ, et al. Obstructive sleep apnea and chronic opioid use. Lung 2010; 188:459–68.

15. Javaheri S, Malik A, Smith J, et al. Adaptive pressure support servoventilation: a novel treatment for sleep apnea associated with use of opioids. J Clin Sleep Med 2008;4:305–10.

16. Dowdell WT, Javaheri S, McGinnis W. Cheyne-Stokes respiration presenting as sleep apnea syndrome: clinical and polysomnographic features. Am Rev Respir Dis 1990;141:871–9.

17. Biot MC. Contribution à l'étude de phénomène respiratoire de Cheyne-Stokes. Lyon Med 1876;23: 561–77 [in French].

18. Javaheri S, Dempsey JA. Central sleep apnea. Compr Physiol 2013;3:141–63.

19. Feldman JL, Del Negro CA. Looking for inspiration: new perspectives on respiratory rhythm. Nat Rev Neurosci 2006;7:232–42.

20. Smith JC, Ellenberger HH, Ballanyi K, et al. Pre-Botzinger complex: a brainstem region that may generate respiratory rhythm in mammals. Science 1991;254:726–9.

21. Montandon G, Qin W, Liu H, et al. PreBotzinger complex neurokinin-1 receptor-expressing neurons mediate opioid-induced respiratory depression. J Neurosci 2011;31:1292–301.

22. Teichtahl H, Wang D, Cunnington D, et al. Ventilatory responses to hypoxia and hypercapnia in stable methadone maintenance treatment patients. Chest 2005;128:1339–47.

23. Ramar K. Reversal of sleep-disordered breathing with opioid withdrawal. Pain Pract 2009;9:394–8.

24. Davis MJ, Livingston M, Scharf SM. Reversal of central sleep apnea following discontinuation of opioids. J Clin Sleep Med 2012;8:579–80.

25. Javaheri S. Heart failure. In: Kryger MH, Roth T, Dement WC, editors. Principles and practice of sleep medicine. 5th edition. Philadelphia: WB Saunders; 2011. p. 1400–15.

26. Glidewell RN, Orr WC, Imes N. Acetazolamide as an adjunct to CPAP treatment: a case of complex sleep apnea in a patient on long-acting opioid therapy. J Clin Sleep Med 2009;5:63–4.

27. Javaheri S. Acetazolamide improves central sleep apnea in heart failure: a double-blind, prospective study. Am J Respir Crit Care Med 2006;173:234–7.

28. Greer JJ, Ren J. Ampakine therapy to counter fentanyl-induced respiratory depression. Respir Physiol Neurobiol 2009;168:153–7.

29. Ren J, Ding X, Funk GD, et al. Ampakine CX717 protects against fentanyl-induced respiratory depression and lethal apnea in rats. Anesthesiology 2009; 110:1364–70.

30. Oertel BG, Felden L, Tran PV, et al. Selective antagonism of opioid-induced ventilatory depression by an ampakine molecule in humans without loss of

opioid analgesia. Clin Pharmacol Ther 2010;87: 204–11.

31. Javaheri S, Smith J, Chung J. The prevalence and natural history of complex sleep apnea. J Clin Sleep Med 2009;5:205–11.

32. Javaheri S. Effects of continuous positive airway pressure on sleep apnea and ventricular irritability in patients with heart failure. Circulation 2000;101: 392–7.

33. Arzt M, Floras JS, Logan AG, et al. Suppression of central sleep apnea by continuous positive airway pressure and transplant-free survival in heart failure. A post-hoc analysis of the Canadian Continuous Positive Airway Pressure for patients with central sleep apnea and heart failure trial (CANPAP). Circulation 2007;115:3173–80.

34. Javaheri S. CPAP should not be used for central sleep apnea in congestive heart failure patients. J Clin Sleep Med 2006;2:399–402.

35. Jilec C, Krenn M, Seha D, et al. Prognostic impact of sleep disordered breathing and its treatment in heart failure: an observational study. Eur J Heart Fail 2011; 13:688–755.

36. Yoshihisa A, Suzuki S, Yamaki T, et al. Impact of adaptive servo-ventilation on cardiovascular function and prognosis in heart failure patients with preserved left ventricular ejection fraction and sleep-disordered breathing. Eur J Heart Fail 2013; 15:543–50.

37. Farney RJ, Walker JM, Boyle KM, et al. Adaptive servoventilation (ASV) in patients with sleep disordered breathing associated with chronic opioid medications for non-malignant pain. J Clin Sleep Med 2008;44:311–9.

38. Allam JS, Olson EJ, Gay PC, et al. Efficacy of adaptive servoventilation in treatment of complex and central sleep apnea syndromes. Chest 2007;132: 1839–46.

39. Alattar MA, Scharf SM. Opioid-associated central sleep apnea: a case series. Sleep Breath 2009;13: 201–6.

40. Harris N, Javaheri S. Advanced positive airway pressure therapy. In: Mattice C, Brooks R, Lee-Chiong T, editors. Fundamentals of sleep technology. Philadelphia: Lippincott Williams & Wilkins; 2012. p. 444–52.

41. Javaheri S, Goetting MG, Khayat R, et al. The performance of two automatic servo-ventilation devices in the treatment of central sleep apnea. Sleep 2011;34: 1693–8.

42. Randerath WJ, Galetke W, Kenter M, et al. Combined adaptive servo-ventilation and automatic positive airway pressure (anticyclic modulated ventilation) in co-existing obstructive and central sleep apnea syndrome and periodic breathing. Sleep Med 2009;10:898–903.

43. Brown LK. Adaptive servo-ventilation for sleep apnea: technology, titration protocols, and treatment efficacy. Sleep Med Clin 2010;5:419–37.

44. Javaheri S. Positive airway pressure treatment of central sleep apnea with emphasis on heart failure, opioids, and complex sleep apnea. In: Berry RB, editor. Sleep medicine clinics. Philadelphia: WB Saunders; 2010. p. 407–17.

45. Ramar K, Ramar P, Morgenthaler TI. Adaptive servo-ventilation in patients with central or complex sleep apnea related to chronic opioid use and congestive heart failure. J Clin Sleep Med 2012;8:569–76.

46. Morganthaler T. The quest for stability in an unstable world: adaptive servoventilation in opioid induced complex sleep apnea syndrome. J Clin Sleep Med 2008;4:311–9.

Central Sleep Apnea due to Other Medical Disorders

Rodrigo Tomazini Martins, MD[a,b], Danny Joel Eckert, PhD[b],*

KEYWORDS

- Sleep-disordered breathing • Lung • Respiratory physiology • Control of breathing
- Respiratory muscles • Neurodegenerative • Neuromuscular

KEY POINTS

- Numerous medical disorders can cause central sleep apnea/hypoventilation.
- This review covers the potential link between brain tumors, Chiari type I malformation, stroke, pain/opioids, endocrine and hormonal disturbances, neurodegenerative disease, neuromuscular disease, and sleep-disordered breathing.
- Control of breathing and potential underlying pathophysiology are highlighted.
- In several medical conditions a bidirectional relationship likely exists whereby the primary medical disorder may cause or worsen central apnea and vice versa.

INTRODUCTION

Central sleep apnea (CSA) is a sleep-related breathing condition characterized by cessation or an evident reduction in airflow lasting at least 10 seconds. Unlike obstructive apnea whereby breathing effort continues but airflow is limited because of upper airway narrowing or collapse, central apneas are associated with absent or insufficient respiratory drive and respiratory muscle output. Similar to obstructive apnea, CSA results in disrupted sleep, frequent arousals, hypercapnia, and hypoxemia.[1,2] CSA is associated with numerous adverse health outcomes including daytime somnolence and cardiovascular disease.[3,4]

There are many manifestations of CSA including the classic crescendo/decrescendo Cheyne-Stokes breathing pattern,[5] common in patients with heart failure. Its presence is associated with poor prognosis. However, certain forms of CSA can also be driven by other pathologic factors. For example, CSA can be caused by damage to the respiratory control centers within the brainstem.[2,6–8]

The most common condition associated with CSA, heart failure,[9] is reviewed elsewhere in this issue in the articles by Caples and Naughton.[10,11] This brief review covers several other medical conditions that may lead to CSA or sleep hypoventilation. The key physiologic components involved in the control of breathing and the reliance on CO_2 to drive ventilation during sleep are highlighted. There follows a brief discussion on a range of medical conditions in which CSA/sleep hypoventilation has been shown to occur, including brain tumors, Chiari type I malformation, stroke, pain/opioids, endocrine and hormonal disturbances (acromegaly, hypothyroidism, pregnancy, metabolic syndrome, diabetes), neurodegenerative disease (multiple sclerosis, multiple-system atrophy, Parkinson disease), and neuromuscular disease

Disclosure Statement: D.J. Eckert is supported by a National Health and Medical Research Council of Australia R.D. Wright Fellowship (1049814). The authors do not have any conflicts of interest to declare in relation to the topic of this article.

[a] Instituto de Neurologia de Curitiba, Neurology Department, Rua Jeremias Maciel Perretto 300, Ecoville, Curitiba, 81210-310, Parana, Brazil; [b] Neuroscience Research Australia (NeuRA), School of Medical Sciences, University of New South Wales, PO Box 1165, Randwick, Sydney, New South Wales 2031, Australia
* Corresponding author.
E-mail address: d.eckert@neura.edu.au

Sleep Med Clin 9 (2014) 57–67
http://dx.doi.org/10.1016/j.jsmc.2013.10.002
1556-407X/14/$ – see front matter © 2014 Elsevier Inc. All rights reserved

(congenital muscular dystrophies, myasthenia gravis, amyotrophic lateral sclerosis). In each case the available evidence linking these various conditions with CSA or sleep hypoventilation are highlighted, and the potential pathophysiologic mechanisms involved are discussed. In many instances a bidirectional relationship likely exists, such that the primary medical condition causes or worsens the CSA while the severity and associated symptoms of the primary medical condition are worsened by the CSA.

PHYSIOLOGY OF CONTROL OF BREATHING AND PATHOPHYSIOLOGY OF CENTRAL SLEEP APNEA
Central Control of Breathing

Neuroanatomically, our understanding of the complex interactions and specific neurons responsible for generating and regulating breathing remains incompletely understood. Primarily based on animal studies, key sites that have been implicated in the central control of breathing within the upper pons include the pontine respiratory group (featuring the nucleus parabrachialis medialis and lateralis, and the Kolliker-Fuse) (**Fig. 1**). These areas have been shown to mediate inspiratory-off phenomena. Lesions above the lower pontine reticular formation cause prolonged inspiratory gasps, and thus are believed to elicit a tonic excitation of inspiratory premotor neurons.[6,7]

Key sites of central respiratory control and rhythmicity, however, lie within the medulla. The dorsal respiratory group, associated with the nucleus tractus solitarius, processes afferent information from phrenic, vagus, and peripheral chemoreceptors to the cortex. This region contains many inspiratory-related neurons, some of which likely mediate inspiratory-off phenomena. It is unclear whether there is direct phrenic output, but nearby projections to the retrotrapezoid nucleus and the ventral respiratory group exist. The ventral respiratory group contains the pre-Bötzinger complex, which has multiple projections to other key brainstem regions involved in the control of breathing.[12] The pre-Bötzinger complex is postulated to be a key pacemaker site, based on the presence of a respiratory rhythm in minimal slice preparations.[13] Conversely, the nearby Bötzinger complex is believed to contribute to expiratory active/inspiratory inhibitory phenomena. The rostral ventral respiratory group contains inspiratory premotor neurons and includes the nucleus ambiguus, which provides motor output to the larynx and pharynx via the vagi.[6,7] **Fig. 1** displays a schematic representation of some of these key sites.

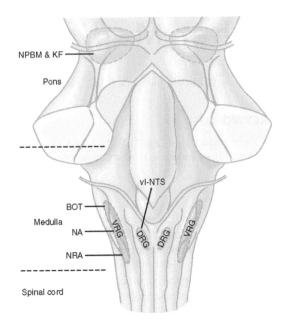

Fig. 1. Central respiratory control centers within the pons and medulla. Refer to the text for further details. BOT, pre-Bötzinger complex; DRG, dorsal respiratory group; KF, Kölliker-Fuse nucleus; NA, nucleus ambiguus; NPBM, nucleus parabrachialis medialis; NRA, nucleus retroambigualis; vl-NTS, ventrolateral nucleus of the tractus solitarius; VRG, ventral respiratory group. (*From* Eckert DJ, Roca D, Yim-Yeh S, et al. Control of breathing. In: Kryger M, editor. Atlas of clinical sleep medicine (2nd edition). Philadelphia: Elsevier Saunders; 2014; with permission.)

Changes in the Inputs to Breathing from Wakefulness to Sleep

During wakefulness, there are multiple inputs that can contribute to the rate and depth at which we breathe, including: cortical voluntary control; emotional input via the limbic system; receptors in muscles and joints; stretch receptors in the lungs; receptors that respond to temperature, pain, and touch; an independent wakefulness drive to breathe; and peripheral chemoreceptors located at the bifurcation of the common carotid arteries.[14] However, the most powerful stimulus to breathe during quiet wakefulness is via the central chemoreceptors.

In reality, virtually all human cells will respond to extreme changes in the surrounding chemical environment. However, certain neurons are exquisitely sensitive to relatively minor changes in the local chemical environment. These areas can either directly regulate the control of breathing or have projections to key central control of breathing sites, and are thus referred to as chemoreceptors. The retrotrapezoid nucleus located on the ventral surface of the medulla adjacent to the ventral respiratory group containing the Bötzinger and pre-Bötzinger neurons has been implicated as a particularly important site of central chemoreception.[15] It responds to partial pressure of CO_2 via changes in the pH of the extracellular fluid. CO_2 diffuses across the blood-brain barrier, increasing the hydrogen ion concentration in the cerebrospinal fluid.

Most inputs capable of regulating breathing during wakefulness are either absent or markedly diminished during sleep. Although chemical control of breathing is also reduced from wakefulness to sleep and changes according to sleep state,[16,17] it becomes the key mediating input for ventilation during sleep (particularly CO_2, as fairly low levels of oxygen are required to stimulate breathing). Our understanding of the relationship between central and peripheral chemoreceptors and the way in which they interact to control breathing continues to evolve.[18] However, the time they respond to local changes in CO_2 varies such that peripheral chemoreceptors are capable of responding within 1 to 2 breaths, whereas central chemoreceptors may take up to a minute. The delays in response time become crucial when considering the pathophysiology of the cyclical breathing patterns associated with CSA.

Pathophysiology of Central Apnea/Sleep Hypoventilation

The pathophysiology of CSA has been reviewed previously,[2,7,19,20] including by Patil elsewhere in this issue.[21] However, the patterns of central breathing instability that occur during sleep can vary considerably between patients and across medical conditions, as does the underlying pathophysiology. This section briefly summarizes the pathophysiologic features that are likely to be important in mediating CSA across different medical conditions. Broadly speaking, central apnea or sleep hypoventilation caused by medical disorders can be due to (1) insufficient drive or interruption in the drive to breathe at the level of the brainstem, or (2) adequate central output from respiratory brainstem neurons, but an inability to translate the central drive to adequate ventilation because of impairment lower down the neuraxis, including respiratory muscle weakness. Some medical disorders may have elements of both of these features. Conceptually the ventilatory control system is regulated by feedback loops. As described earlier, CO_2 is the key modulator of the ventilatory control system during sleep. The respiratory feedback loop can be described by the engineering term loop gain.[7,22,23] The three key components

of loop gain are: 1) plant gain (efficiency of breathing to excrete CO_2 as determined by the characteristics of the lungs, blood, and body tissues), 2) mixing and circulation delays (the time required for a change in CO_2 to mix with the existing blood in the heart and the arteries before reaching the chemoreceptors), and 3) controller gain (chemoresponsiveness; eg, hypercapnic ventilatory response). If a disease state alters one or more of these elements (eg, lung volume is reduced or chemoreceptor sensitivity is heightened) it can lead to a high loop gain state and cyclical breathing instability can ensue. While increased circulation delay in of itself doesn't increase loop gain per se, it is important in determining the length and duration of breathing instability. As highlighted below, without circulation delay cyclical breathing instability would not occur.

Other physiological processes that are important in contributing to CSA include state instability,[7] the ventilatory response to arousal[24,25] and the apnea threshold.[26] During the transition from wakefulness to sleep many excitatory inputs to breathing are rapidly removed including the wakefulness drive to breathe.[14] If the loss of these inputs is substantial, central apneas can occur. Indeed, central apneas do occur quite commonly even in otherwise healthy individuals during the transition from wakefulness to sleep. During sleep, transient awakenings (cortical arousals) lead to a brisk increase in breathing.[24] This causes a relative state of hypocapnia upon the resumption of sleep. If the change is large or an individual is particularly sensitive to relatively small fluctuations in CO_2 during sleep, as is the case in certain disease states,[27] the apnea threshold may be crossed leading to central apnea. The apnea threshold reflects a critical level of CO_2 below which there is insufficient drive to breathe.[26] This value varies between individuals and across disease states but is often only a few Torr below the stable sleeping CO_2 level. Given that it takes time for the ventilatory control feedback system to respond to sudden changes in CO_2 (due to circulation delays), rapid reductions in CO_2 can therefore lead to breathing cessation.[25,28]

MEDICAL DISORDERS ASSOCIATED WITH CENTRAL SLEEP APNEA

As already mentioned, the most common medical cause of CSA is heart failure.[29] The high prevalence of this comorbidity is still underrecognized, but CSA may be present in up to 70% of patients with heart failure, especially males.[30] This section covers other medical disorders in which CSA typically occurs less frequently than in heart failure, but when present is likely to further perpetuate adverse health outcomes and the consequences of the primary medical condition. Understanding the underlying pathophysiology is crucial in attempting to treat CSA in these patients, which can often be challenging.

Renal Failure

Patients with renal failure on hemodialysis often experience poor sleep and are affected by obstructive, central, and mixed apnea at higher rates than occur in the general population.[6] These patients usually have comorbidities such as heart failure, diabetes, and stroke. Many systems may be affected by these conditions, making it difficult to determine the exact pathophysiology responsible for mediating the CSA.[31]

It is postulated that hydro-overload and fluid-volume redistribution during the decubitus state cause edema of the upper airway, leading to obstructive apnea.[32,33] Regarding CSA, these patients frequently present with increased uremia, inducing a state of acidosis and hypocapnia accompanied by increased chemosensitivity.[31,34] This process increases loop gain and the potential to cross the apnea threshold during sleep. Fluid accumulation may also affect respiratory afferents and cause inhibition of breathing.[35] State instability may play a further role in contributing to periodic breathing instability in these patients, who often have difficulty obtaining deeper sleep. The population most affected by renal failure and CSA are male, older, and have a high body mass index.[34]

Brain Tumors

Among the pediatric population referred to a sleep clinic who are affected by brain tumors, up to 90% involve tumors located within brainstem, thalamus, or hypothalamus.[36] In addition to daytime sleepiness, tumors in these locations can often cause respiratory irregularities during sleep when wakefulness-determined behavioral compensatory mechanisms are lost. Of the few reported cases of CSA involving tumors in this population, tumors have been located in the brainstem, fourth ventricle, posterior fossa, and spinal region. Thus, dysfunction or interruption of respiratory neural output at multiple sites within the central nervous system may cause CSA. Unlike patients with tumors and obstructive sleep apnea who are often also obese, CSA patients tend to be nonobese.[37]

In adults, CSA may occur in the presence of brain tumors[38–40] or following their surgical resection.[39,41,42] Direct compression from the tumor itself, hemorrhage, or surrounding edema caused by the lesions, may impair brainstem respiratory control centers (**Fig. 2**). Areas such as the reticular formation, nucleus ambiguus, and solitary tract have been implicated.[40] Impairment of these regions may lead to blunted chemosensitivity and hypercapnia caused by diminished ventilatory output, leading to hypoventilation during sleep and CSA.[7]

Chiari Type I Malformation

Chiari type I malformation is associated with both obstructive apnea and CSA, affecting pediatric and adult populations. CSA and hypoventilation can be present in both rapid eye movement (REM) and non-REM (NREM) sleep. The extent of the malformation present and the downstream effects on control of breathing centers vary between patients (eg, **Fig. 3**). However, polysomnography changes correlate well with magnetic resonance imaging (MRI) findings.[43,44] CSA tends to be more severe in children who present with syrinx and general crowding at the foramen magnum.[43–45]

Possible mechanisms by which Chiari type I malformation is believed to cause CSA include compression of pre-Bötzinger neurons leading to

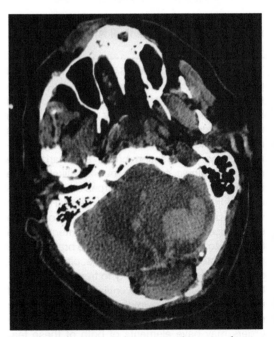

Fig. 2. Axial computed tomography scan from a 67-year-old man with a history of smoking, chronic obstructive pulmonary disease, snoring, and apnea, particularly during rapid eye movement (REM) sleep. Postsurgical status showing a posterior fossa tumor evolving with hemorrhage, and massive edema compressing the pons ventrally.

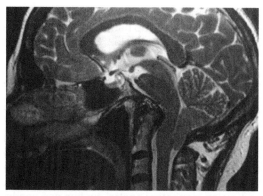

Fig. 3. Sagittal T1-weighted magnetic resonance image of a 42-year-old woman with Chiari type I malformation. Ectopic cerebellar tonsil insinuates through the foramen magnum, with dorsal compression to the cervicomedullary transition and ventral compression by odontoid process. Cerebellar tonsil herniation measured 1.3 cm below the foramen magnum.

dysfunction of respiratory centers, medullary compression and local ischemia, and altered chemoreceptor function. These impediments to breathing are often overcome during wakefulness, but can result in CSA during sleep when compensatory wakefulness mechanisms are absent. Decompression of the affected regions has been shown to reduce or eliminate the sleep-disordered breathing.

Stroke

Snoring is associated with a higher risk of developing cerebrovascular disease (transient ischemic attack or stroke). Cerebrovascular disease is also a risk factor for CSA, especially in cases with brainstem involvement.[46–48] Thus, there is likely a bidirectional relationship between stroke and sleep-disordered breathing. In many cases the classic crescendo/decrescendo Cheyne-Stokes breathing pattern is present. Indeed, the initial report of this breathing pattern was based on observations in a patient with both stroke and congestive heart failure.[5]

CSA is common in patients with cerebral microangiopathy, supratentorial strokes, or brainstem lesions, particularly in the immediate poststroke period. Whereas CSA may resolve over time in some patients, many seem to retain CSA even when otherwise stable.[49] Associations between loss of cerebral white matter and CSA have been reported.[50] In an elegant recently published study, Duning and colleagues[51] used a range of detailed MRI techniques, including diffusion tensor imaging, in patients with Fabry disease as a model for microangiopathy, some of whom also had CSA.

In the CSA patients, the investigators were able to detect subtle changes in microstructural neural networks within the brainstem, and the severity of CSA correlated with structural brainstem damage as measured by diffusion tensor imaging.[51] Although it is not precisely clear how these changes affect respiratory control (ie, altered chemosensitivity[48] or a direct effect on control of breathing centers, or both), these findings do suggest that even relatively subtle changes in these brainstem regions can lead to CSA.

Pain and Opioids

The effect of drugs in CSA is reviewed elsewhere in this issue by Javaheri,[52] and thus is only covered briefly here. It is clear that opioid receptors are located diversely within the central and peripheral nervous systems and, in addition to affecting nociception, are capable of affecting respiratory neurons. Opioid analgesic prescriptions are becoming more frequent in pain clinical practice, and may contribute to sleep-related breathing disorders. However, their effect is likely to be highly dose dependent. Mild doses may have minimal effect on sleep and breathing, moderate doses may manifest as intermittent pauses in breathing during sleep (effectively when central pattern generator neurons transiently do not fire), and higher doses are more likely to cause CSA and sustained hypoventilation.[7,53–55] Opioid-induced changes in chemosensitivity at higher doses likely play a key contributing role in CSA.[56] Poor sleep quality can worsen pain, and pain can lead to poor sleep quality.[57] Accordingly, analgesic requirements may further increase worsening sleep to create a vicious circular cycle. Alternatively, if the balance is optimized, low doses of opioids may improve pain and sleep, although this concept has been minimally studied.[58]

Endocrine and Hormonal Disturbances

Acromegaly

Obstructive apnea is common in patients with acromegaly. However, CSA is also common in these patients.[59,60] Compared with healthy controls and acromegaly patients with obstructive apnea, the presence of CSA in acromegaly is associated with increased serum levels of growth hormone and insulin-like growth factor 1, and heightened ventilatory responsiveness to CO_2.[60] Elevated chemosensitivity increases loop gain and, thus, the propensity toward CSA.

Hypothyroidism

Hypothyroidism has been implicated in sleep-disordered breathing, and changes in respiratory control have been postulated to be a contributing mechanism.[59,61] However, there is little evidence to support a potential causal link between CSA and hypothyroidism. In a case report,[62] a blunted neuromuscular and ventilatory response to hypoxia was observed without diminished responsiveness to CO_2 in a middle-aged patient with hypothyroidism and CSA. Hormone replacement with levothyroxine was successful in alleviating the CSA and restoring the hypoxic ventilatory response.

Pregnancy

A range of physiologic and hormonal changes take place throughout pregnancy. Some of these changes may contribute to sleep-disordered breathing, whereas others are likely to be protective.[63–65] For example, increased body weight, edema (including nasopharyngeal), cranial displacement of the diaphragm, and reduced lung volume may each contribute to sleep-disordered breathing. Conversely, increased progesterone likely plays a protective role by increasing minute ventilation.[63–65] Thus, the presence or absence of sleep-disordered breathing in pregnancy depends on a range of complex physiologic interactions. Nonetheless, snoring and obstructive sleep apnea is common during mid to late pregnancy. The link between CSA and pregnancy is less clear, but cases have been reported.[66] Conceptually, increased loop gain via lung-volume reduction,[67] inhibitory effects associated with edema,[35] or sleep-state instability attributable to increased lighter sleep[68] may contribute to CSA in pregnancy. However, these effects would have to outweigh the opposing protective respiratory stimulant effects of progesterone, which would tend to lower plant gain and, therefore, overall loop gain.

Other endocrine or hormonal disturbances

There are clear links between metabolic syndrome, diabetes, sleep disruption, and sleep-disordered breathing.[59,69–72] Most commonly the presence of obesity in patients with metabolic syndrome and diabetes has been implicated as a cause of obstructive apnea. However, similar to mass loading of the abdomen in pregnancy, central obesity may also decrease lung volume during sleep, particularly in the supine posture.[73] Accordingly, loop gain and the propensity for CSA increase.[67] Ventilatory control may also be affected in these conditions, although this has been minimally studied.

Hormones such as testosterone have been shown to increase chemosensitivity and the apnea threshold.[74,75] Thus, testosterone may increase the propensity for CSA in men. Conversely, estrogens and progestins may play a protective role by widening the gap between eupneic breathing and the apnea threshold.[76]

Neurodegenerative Diseases

Multiple sclerosis

Sleep disturbances and fatigue are common in patients with multiple sclerosis.[77] MS patients presenting with brainstem involvement documented through neuroimaging are twice as likely to display CSA, particularly in those with progressive subtypes caused by scattering parenchymal injury embracing respiratory control centers and nearby brainstem precincts. Demyelinating plaques at the medullary reticular formation may cause impaired respiratory control. It is currently unclear whether midbrain, pontine, or medullary locations are more associated with the severity of CSA in patients with MS.[78] Respiratory muscle weakness occurs in the later stages of MS,[79] and may also contribute to CSA.

Multiple-system atrophy

Almost all patients with multiple-system atrophy have REM behavior disorder and stridor, characterized by its high-pitched tone. These features typically appear well before waking motor and dysautonomic onset. Although obstructive apnea is more common, CSA can occur as the primary presenting issue in multiple-system atrophy.[80,81] However, CSA tends to occur more often in the advanced stages of the disease.[82–84] When present, CSA in multiple-system atrophy may manifest in a variety of forms including Cheyne-Stokes breathing or other forms of dysrhythmic breathing.[82] Medullary serotonergic neurons are depleted in multiple-system atrophy.[85] Postmortem inspection of brainstem slices from patients with multiple-system atrophy has also revealed widespread damage to respiratory chemoreceptive neurons, particularly in the ventral medullary surface.[86] Thus, impaired function of central chemoreceptors is likely to be a key contributing factor to CSA in patients with multiple-system atrophy. More recently, pre-Bötzinger complex neurons have been shown to be reduced in these patients,[8,87] an effect that is likely to play a key role in the development of CSA.

Parkinson disease

Sleep-disordered breathing affects up to 40% of patients with Parkinson disease. There is a predominance of obstructive sleep apnea; however, central apneas can also occur, predominantly in male patients.[83,88,89] Neurochemical deficits in Parkinson disease are complex. Using positron emission tomography imaging, Lelieveld and colleagues[88] investigated the potential link between impairment of caudal brainstem serotoninergic and striatal dopaminergic innervation and sleep-disordered breathing. No association was observed, suggesting that other neuromodulator systems (eg, cholinergic and noradrenergic) may be involved. It is also possible that dopamine agonists used in the management of Parkinson disease may alter respiratory control[90] and might contribute to breathing instability during sleep, although this has been minimally studied.

Neuromuscular Disease

Congenital muscular dystrophies

Congenital muscular dystrophies are inherited diseases affecting muscles. In addition to poor-quality sleep and seizures, sleep-disordered breathing is present in approximately 65% of cases.[91–94] CSA is the most common form of sleep-related breathing instability in patients with congenital muscular dystrophies.[92] The severity of CSA is related to the age of onset of symptoms and the rate of progression of muscle weakness.[92] The primary mechanism by which CSA occurs in these patients is via an inability to translate respiratory neural drive from the respiratory centers (which may be perfectly normal) into functional motion of the respiratory muscles, because of muscle weakness. Whereas in some of these patients a degree of hypoventilation can occur during wakefulness leading to CO_2 retention, others remain normocapnic, with hypoventilation only occurring during sleep when wakefulness neuro-compensatory mechanisms are lost. Thus, unlike other forms of CSA that typically worsen in NREM sleep, CSA in patients with congenital muscular dystrophies may be most pronounced during REM sleep against the background of already low drive to the intercostal muscles and accessory respiratory muscles.[92,95] Poor sleep quality may also perpetuate state-stability CSA in these patients.

Myasthenia gravis

Myasthenia gravis, an autoimmune condition characterized by antibodies inactivating acetylcholine receptors at the neuromuscular junction, is associated with sleep-disordered breathing even when patients are medically stable. However, whereas some studies report a predominance of central apneas, others report obstructive apnea being more common.[96–98] Respiratory muscle weakness is the key contributing mechanism to CSA in these patients, with REM predominance.

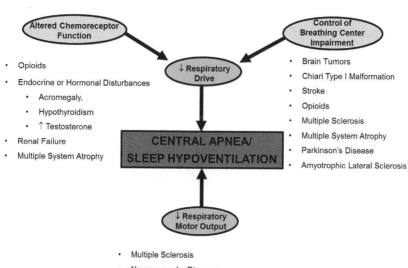

Fig. 4. Potential pathophysiologic factors contributing to central sleep apnea/sleep hypoventilation caused by medical disorders. Sleep-state instability (common in many of these conditions) may also cause or worsen existing sleep-disordered breathing. Medical disorders in which decreased respiratory drive is the predominating cause will tend to be worse in lighter non-REM sleep, whereas disorders affecting respiratory motor output will tend to be worse in REM sleep. For simplicity, several potential contributing mechanisms are not represented. Refer to the text for further details.

Amyotrophic lateral sclerosis

Amyotrophic lateral sclerosis is a neurodegenerative disease characterized by progressive paralysis caused by motoneuron degeneration of bulbar, diaphragmatic, and intercostal muscles.[6] Death from respiratory failure typically occurs within years. Sleep-disordered breathing may reflect an early abnormality attributable to ALS.[83,93,99,100] Respiratory muscle weakness leading to hypoventilation, particularly during REM sleep, is common. Motoneurons affecting central respiratory control may also be affected in this disease.[99]

SUMMARY

Numerous medical disorders can lead to CSA or sleep hypoventilation (**Fig. 4**). Disorders that affect respiratory control centers or chemoreceptor function can lead to inadequate drive to breathe during sleep when wakefulness neurocompensatory mechanisms are absent. A diminished ability to translate central respiratory drive into adequate ventilation can also be caused by pathologic conditions arising from impairment lower down the neuraxis, including respiratory muscle weakness. Some medical disorders may have dysfunction on multiple levels (see **Fig. 4**). A bidirectional relationship likely exists for many of these conditions, such that the primary medical disorder causes or worsens the CSA and its adverse effects while the primary medical condition and its associated symptoms are worsened by the CSA. There is a need to explore these relationships and improve the understanding of the underlying mechanisms mediating the link between certain medical conditions and CSA, and the potential to intervene to improve health outcomes.

REFERENCES

1. Malhotra A, Owens RL. What is central sleep apnea? Respir Care 2010;55:1168–78.
2. Eckert DJ, Malhotra A, Jordan AS. Mechanisms of apnea. Prog Cardiovasc Dis 2009;51:313–23.
3. Khayat R, Abraham W, Patt B, et al. Central sleep apnea is a predictor of cardiac readmission in hospitalized patients with systolic heart failure. J Card Fail 2012;18:534–40.
4. Bakker JP, Campbell AJ, Neill AM. Increased mortality risk in congestive heart failure patients with comorbid sleep apnoea: 10-year follow up. Intern Med J 2012;42:1264–8.
5. Cheyne J. A case of apoplexy in which the fleshy part of the heart was converted into fat. Dublin Hosp Rep 1818;2:216–23.
6. Kehlmann GB, Eckert DJ. Central sleep apnea due to a medical condition not Cheyne Stokes. In: Kushida CA, editor. Encyclopedia of sleep. San Diego (CA): Elsevier; 2013. p. 244–52.
7. Eckert DJ, Jordan AS, Merchia P, et al. Central sleep apnea: pathophysiology and treatment. Chest 2007;131:595–607.
8. Schwarzacher SW, Rub U, Deller T. Neuroanatomical characteristics of the human pre-Bötzinger complex and its involvement in neurodegenerative brainstem diseases. Brain 2011; 134:24–35.
9. Yumino D, Kasai T, Kimmerly D, et al. Differing effects of obstructive and central sleep apneas on stroke volume in patients with heart failure. Am J Respir Crit Care Med 2013;187:433–8.
10. Caples S. Central sleep apnea and cardiovascular disease. Sleep Med Clin.
11. Naughton MT. Cheyne-Stokes respiration. Sleep Med Clin.
12. Tan W, Pagliardini S, Yang P, et al. Projections of pre-Bötzinger complex neurons in adult rats. J Comp Neurol 2010;518:1862–78.
13. Smith JC, Ellenberger HH, Ballanyi K, et al. Pre-Bötzinger complex: a brainstem region that may generate respiratory rhythm in mammals. Science 1991;254:726–9.
14. Eckert DJ, Roca D, Yim-Yeh S, et al. Control of breathing. In: Kryger M, editor. Atlas of clinical sleep medicine. 2nd edition. Philadelphia: Elsevier Saunders; 2014. p. 45–52.
15. Wang S, Shi Y, Shu S, et al. Phox2b-expressing retrotrapezoid neurons are intrinsically responsive to H^+ and CO_2. J Neurosci 2013;33:7756–61.
16. Douglas NJ, White DP, Weil JV, et al. Hypoxic ventilatory response decreases during sleep in normal men. Am Rev Respir Dis 1982;125:286–9.
17. Douglas NJ, White DP, Weil JV, et al. Hypercapnic ventilatory response in sleeping adults. Am Rev Respir Dis 1982;126:758–62.
18. Dempsey JA, Smith CA, Blain GM, et al. Role of central/peripheral chemoreceptors and their interdependence in the pathophysiology of sleep apnea. Adv Exp Med Biol 2012;758:343–9.
19. McSharry DG, Eckert DJ, Malhotra A. Central sleep apnoea. In: McNicholas WT, Bonsignore MR, editors. Sleep apnoea: European Respiratory Society monograph, vol. 50. Plymouth (United Kingdom): ERS Educational Publications; 2010. p. 381–95.
20. Javaheri S. Central sleep apnea. Clin Chest Med 2010;31:235–48.
21. Patil SP. Mechanisms and pathophysiology of central sleep apnea. Sleep Med Clin.
22. Khoo MC, Gottschalk A, Pack AI. Sleep-induced periodic breathing and apnea: a theoretical study. J Appl Phys 1991;70:2014–24.
23. Khoo MC, Kronauer RE, Strohl KP, et al. Factors inducing periodic breathing in humans: a general model. J Appl Phys 1982;53:644–59.

24. Jordan AS, Eckert DJ, Catcheside PG, et al. Ventilatory response to brief arousal from non-rapid eye movement sleep is greater in men than in women. Am J Respir Crit Care Med 2003;168:1512–9.

25. Khoo MC, Koh SS, Shin JJ, et al. Ventilatory dynamics during transient arousal from NREM sleep: implications for respiratory control stability. J Appl Phys 1996;80:1475–84.

26. Dempsey JA. Crossing the apnoeic threshold: causes and consequences. Exp Physiol 2005;90:13–24.

27. Xie A, Skatrud JB, Puleo DS, et al. Apnea-hypopnea threshold for CO_2 in patients with congestive heart failure. Am J Respir Crit Care Med 2002;165:1245–50.

28. Xie A, Wong B, Phillipson EA, et al. Interaction of hyperventilation and arousal in the pathogenesis of idiopathic central sleep apnea. Am J Respir Crit Care Med 1994;150:489–95.

29. Cao M, Guilleminault C, Lin C. Central sleep apnea: effects on stroke volume in heart failure. Am J Respir Crit Care Med 2013;187:340–1.

30. Oldenburg O. Cheyne-Stokes respiration in chronic heart failure. Treatment with adaptive servoventilation therapy. Circ J 2012;76:2305–17.

31. Tang SC, Lai KN. Sleep disturbances and sleep apnea in patients on chronic peritoneal dialysis. J Nephrol 2009;22:318–25.

32. Elias RM, Bradley TD, Kasai T, et al. Rostral overnight fluid shift in end-stage renal disease: relationship with obstructive sleep apnea. Nephrol Dial Transplant 2012;27:1569–73.

33. Elias RM, Chan CT, Paul N, et al. Relationship of pharyngeal water content and jugular volume with severity of obstructive sleep apnea in renal failure. Nephrol Dial Transplant 2013;28:937–44.

34. Beecroft J, Duffin J, Pierratos A, et al. Enhanced chemo-responsiveness in patients with sleep apnoea and end-stage renal disease. Eur Respir J 2006;28:151–8.

35. Pisarri TE, Jonzon A, Coleridge HM, et al. Vagal afferent and reflex responses to changes in surface osmolarity in lower airways of dogs. J Appl Phys 1992;73:2305–13.

36. Rosen GM, Shor AC, Geller TJ. Sleep in children with cancer. Curr Opin Pediatr 2008;20:676–81.

37. Mandrell BN, Wise M, Schoumacher RA, et al. Excessive daytime sleepiness and sleep-disordered breathing disturbances in survivors of childhood central nervous system tumors. Pediatr Blood Cancer 2012;58:746–51.

38. Valente S, De Rosa M, Culla G, et al. An uncommon case of brainstem tumor with selective involvement of the respiratory centers. Chest 1993;103:1909–10.

39. Manning HL, Leiter JC. Respiratory control and respiratory sensation in a patient with a ganglioglioma within the dorsocaudal brain stem. Am J Respir Crit Care Med 2000;161:2100–6.

40. Maiuri F, Esposito M. Positional and sleep dyspnoea due to posterior exophytic ependymoma of the medulla oblongata. J Neurol Neurosurg Psychiatr 2005;76:804.

41. Matsuyama M, Nakazawa K, Katou M, et al. Central alveolar hypoventilation syndrome due to surgical resection for bulbar hemangioblastoma. Intern Med 2009;48:925–30.

42. Afaq T, Magalang UJ, Das AM. An unusual cause of insomnia. Central sleep apnea (CSA). J Clin Sleep Med 2012;8:623–5.

43. Dhamija R, Wetjen NM, Slocumb NL, et al. The role of nocturnal polysomnography in assessing children with Chiari type I malformation. Clin Neurol Neurosurg 2013;115(9):1837–41.

44. Khatwa U, Ramgopal S, Mylavarapu A, et al. MRI findings and sleep apnea in children with Chiari I malformation. Pediatr Neurol 2013;48:299–307.

45. Addo NK, Javadpour S, Kandasamy J, et al. Central sleep apnea and associated Chiari malformation in children with syndromic craniosynostosis: treatment and outcome data from a supraregional national craniofacial center. J Neurosurg Pediatr 2013;11:296–301.

46. Valham F, Mooe T, Rabben T, et al. Increased risk of stroke in patients with coronary artery disease and sleep apnea: a 10-year follow-up. Circ J 2008;118:955–60.

47. Bonnin-Vilaplana M, Arboix A, Parra O, et al. Cheyne-Stokes respiration in patients with first-ever lacunar stroke. Sleep Disord 2012;2012:257890.

48. Rupprecht S, Hoyer D, Hagemann G, et al. Central sleep apnea indicates autonomic dysfunction in asymptomatic carotid stenosis: a potential marker of cerebrovascular and cardiovascular risk. Sleep 2010;33:327–33.

49. Sacchetti ML, Di Mascio MT, Fiorelli M, et al. Post stroke sleep apnea hypopnea syndrome: a series of 12 consecutive stable stroke cases. Eur Rev Med Pharmacol Sci 2012;16:1295–300.

50. Robbins J, Redline S, Ervin A, et al. Associations of sleep-disordered breathing and cerebral changes on MRI. J Clin Sleep Med 2005;1:159–65.

51. Duning T, Deppe M, Brand E, et al. Brainstem involvement as a cause of central sleep apnea: pattern of microstructural cerebral damage in patients with cerebral microangiopathy. PLoS One 2013;8:e60304.

52. Javaheri S. Drug induced central apneas—mechanism and therapies. Sleep Med Clin.

53. Wang D, Eckert DJ, Grunstein RR. Drug effects on ventilatory control and upper airway physiology related to sleep apnea. Respir Physiolo Neurobiol 2013;188(3):257–66.

54. Wang D, Somogyi AA, Yee BJ, et al. The effects of a single mild dose of morphine on chemoreflexes and breathing in obstructive sleep apnea. Respir Physiolo Neurobiol 2013;185:526–32.

55. Wang D, Teichtahl H, Drummer O, et al. Central sleep apnea in stable methadone maintenance treatment patients. Chest 2005;128:1348–56.

56. Teichtahl H, Wang D, Cunnington D, et al. Ventilatory responses to hypoxia and hypercapnia in stable methadone maintenance treatment patients. Chest 2005;128:1339–47.

57. Panagiotou I, Mystakidou K. Non-analgesic effects of opioids: opioids' effects on sleep (including sleep apnea). Curr Pharm Des 2012;18:6025–33.

58. Brennan MJ, Lieberman JA 3rd. Sleep disturbances in patients with chronic pain: effectively managing opioid analgesia to improve outcomes. Curr Med Res Opin 2009;25:1045–55.

59. Bottini P, Tantucci C. Sleep apnea syndrome in endocrine diseases. Respiration 2003;70:320–7.

60. Grunstein RR, Ho KY, Berthon-Jones M, et al. Central sleep apnea is associated with increased ventilatory response to carbon dioxide and hypersecretion of growth hormone in patients with acromegaly. Am J Respir Crit Care Med 1994; 150:496–502.

61. Rosenow F, McCarthy V, Caruso AC. Sleep apnoea in endocrine diseases. J Sleep Res 1998;7:3–11.

62. Millman RP, Bevilacqua J, Peterson DD, et al. Central sleep apnea in hypothyroidism. Am Rev Respir Dis 1983;127:504–7.

63. Venkata C, Venkateshiah SB. Sleep-disordered breathing during pregnancy. J Am Board Fam Med 2009;22:158–68.

64. Elkus R, Popovich J Jr. Respiratory physiology in pregnancy. Clin Chest Med 1992;13:555–65.

65. Contreras G, Gutierrez M, Beroiza T, et al. Ventilatory drive and respiratory muscle function in pregnancy. Am Rev Respir Dis 1991;144:837–41.

66. Ochoa-Sepulveda JJ, Ochoa-Amor JJ. Ondine's curse during pregnancy. J Neurol Neurosurg Psychiatr 2005;76:294.

67. Edwards BA, Sands SA, Feeney C, et al. Continuous positive airway pressure reduces loop gain and resolves periodic central apneas in the lamb. Respir Physiolo Neurobiol 2009;168:239–49.

68. Pien GW, Schwab RJ. Sleep disorders during pregnancy. Sleep 2004;27:1405–17.

69. Saaresranta T, Polo O. Sleep-disordered breathing and hormones. Eur Respir J 2003;22:161–72.

70. Hall MH, Okun ML, Sowers M, et al. Sleep is associated with the metabolic syndrome in a multiethnic cohort of midlife women: the SWAN Sleep Study. Sleep 2012;35:783–90.

71. Gasa M, Salord N, Fortuna AM, et al. Obstructive sleep apnoea and metabolic impairment in severe obesity. Eur Respir J 2011;38:1089–97.

72. Sanders MH, Givelber R. Sleep disordered breathing may not be an independent risk factor for diabetes, but diabetes may contribute to the occurrence of periodic breathing in sleep. Sleep Med 2003;4:349–50.

73. Stadler DL, McEvoy RD, Sprecher KE, et al. Abdominal compression increases upper airway collapsibility during sleep in obese male obstructive sleep apnea patients. Sleep 2009;32: 1579–87.

74. Zhou XS, Rowley JA, Demirovic F, et al. Effect of testosterone on the apneic threshold in women during NREM sleep. J Appl Phys 2003;94:101–7.

75. Ahuja D, Mateika JH, Diamond MP, et al. Ventilatory sensitivity to carbon dioxide before and after episodic hypoxia in women treated with testosterone. J Appl Phys 2007;102:1832–8.

76. Rowley JA, Zhou XS, Diamond MP, et al. The determinants of the apnea threshold during NREM sleep in normal subjects. Sleep 2006;29:95–103.

77. Kaminska M, Kimoff RJ, Schwartzman K, et al. Sleep disorders and fatigue in multiple sclerosis: evidence for association and interaction. J Neurol Sci 2011;302:7–13.

78. Braley TJ, Segal BM, Chervin RD. Sleep-disordered breathing in multiple sclerosis. Neurology 2012;79:929–36.

79. Gosselink R, Kovacs L, Decramer M. Respiratory muscle involvement in multiple sclerosis. Eur Respir J 1999;13:449–54.

80. Cormican LJ, Higgins S, Davidson AC, et al. Multiple system atrophy presenting as central sleep apnoea. Eur Respir J 2004;24:323–5.

81. Glass GA, Josephs KA, Ahlskog JE. Respiratory insufficiency as the primary presenting symptom of multiple-system atrophy. Arch Neurol 2006;63: 978–81.

82. Ferini-Strambi L, Marelli S. Sleep dysfunction in multiple system atrophy. Curr Treat Options Neurol 2012;14:464–73.

83. Gaig C, Iranzo A. Sleep-disordered breathing in neurodegenerative diseases. Curr Neurol Neurosci Rep 2012;12:205–17.

84. Iranzo A. Sleep and breathing in multiple system atrophy. Curr Treat Options Neurol 2007;9:347–53.

85. Tada M, Kakita A, Toyoshima Y, et al. Depletion of medullary serotonergic neurons in patients with multiple system atrophy who succumbed to sudden death. Brain 2009;132:1810–9.

86. Benarroch EE, Schmeichel AM, Low PA, et al. Depletion of putative chemosensitive respiratory neurons in the ventral medullary surface in multiple system atrophy. Brain 2007;130:469–75.

87. Ramirez JM. The human pre-Bötzinger complex identified. Brain 2011;134:8–10.

88. Lelieveld IM, Muller ML, Bohnen NI, et al. The role of serotonin in sleep disordered breathing

associated with Parkinson disease: a correlative [^{11}C]DASB PET imaging study. PLoS One 2012;7: e40166.

89. Maria B, Sophia S, Michalis M, et al. Sleep breathing disorders in patients with idiopathic Parkinson's disease. Respir Med 2003;97:1151–7.

90. Lalley PM. D1/D2-dopamine receptor agonist dihydrexidine stimulates inspiratory motor output and depresses medullary expiratory neurons. Am J Physiol Regul Integr Comp Physiol 2009;296: R1829–36.

91. Quijano-Roy S, Galan L, Ferreiro A, et al. Severe progressive form of congenital muscular dystrophy with calf pseudohypertrophy, macroglossia and respiratory insufficiency. Neuromuscul Disord 2002;12:466–75.

92. Pinard JM, Azabou E, Essid N, et al. Sleep-disordered breathing in children with congenital muscular dystrophies. Europ J Paediatr Neurol 2012;16:619–24.

93. Labanowski M, Schmidt-Nowara W, Guilleminault C. Sleep and neuromuscular disease: frequency of sleep-disordered breathing in a neuromuscular disease clinic population. Neurology 1996;47:1173–80.

94. Kryger MH, Steljes DG, Yee WC, et al. Central sleep apnoea in congenital muscular dystrophy. J Neurol Neurosurg Psychiatr 1991;54:710–2.

95. Suresh S, Wales P, Dakin C, et al. Sleep-related breathing disorder in Duchenne muscular dystrophy: disease spectrum in the paediatric population. J Paediatr Child Health 2005;41:500–3.

96. Amino A, Shiozawa Z, Nagasaka T, et al. Sleep apnoea in well-controlled myasthenia gravis and the effect of thymectomy. J Neurol 1998;245:77–80.

97. Quera-Salva MA, Guilleminault C, Chevret S, et al. Breathing disorders during sleep in myasthenia gravis. Ann Neurol 1992;31:86–92.

98. Prudlo J, Koenig J, Ermert S, et al. Sleep disordered breathing in medically stable patients with myasthenia gravis. Eur J Neurol 2007;14:321–6.

99. Atalaia A, De Carvalho M, Evangelista T, et al. Sleep characteristics of amyotrophic lateral sclerosis in patients with preserved diaphragmatic function. Amyotroph Lateral Scler 2007;8:101–5.

100. Katzberg HD, Selegiman A, Guion L, et al. Effects of noninvasive ventilation on sleep outcomes in amyotrophic lateral sclerosis. J Clin Sleep Med 2013;9:345–51.

Adaptive Servoventilation in Central Sleep Apnea

Winfried J. Randerath, MD[a],*, Shahrokh Javaheri, MD[b]

KEYWORDS

- Adaptive servoventilation • Cheyne-Stokes respiration • Central sleep apnea
- Positive airway pressure

KEY POINTS

- There is increasing evidence that central sleep apnea and Cheyne-Stokes respiration are associated with a poor prognosis in patients with heart failure.
- Continuous positive airway pressure (CPAP), bilevel positive airway pressure (BPAP) and oxygen might reduce, but not normalize central sleep apnea/Cheyne-Stokes respiration CSA/CSR in heart failure.
- Optimal suppression of respiratory disturbances is crucial to improve outcome of patients with cardiovascular diseases.
- Adaptive servoventilation counterbalances ventilatory over- and undershoot and is superior to other PAP treatments or oxygen.
- Open questions include the influence of ASV on survival of heart failure patients and its use in other phenotypes of CSA.

INTRODUCTION

Since the description of effective treatment of the obstructive sleep apnea syndrome (OSAS) with continuous positive airway pressure (CPAP),[1] the awareness of sleep-related breathing disorders (SRBDs) has risen rapidly in the medical community. An increasing number of patients with severe underlying comorbidities, including cardiovascular diseases, renal failure, and neurologic disorders, are presenting to sleep laboratories. This trend has led to growing recognition obstructive phenotypes other than breathing disturbances during sleep. Obstructive sleep apnea (OSA) has to be separated from hypocapnic and hypercapnic central breathing disturbances. Whereas hypocapnic disturbances are characterized by hyperventilation resulting in a diminished arterial pressure of carbon dioxide ($PaCO_2$), the respiratory drive is reduced in hypercapnia. Idiopathic central sleep apnea (ICSA) and Cheyne-Stokes respiration (CSR) are typical representations of hypocapnic central sleep apnea (CSA). Opioid-induced CSA and obesity-related hypoventilation represent hypercapnic central disturbances.[2,3]

As arousals, hypoxemia, and breathing effort can increase sympathoadrenal activity, SRBDs impair heart function. The left ventricular transmural pressure (ie, the afterload) is increased.[4,5] In addition, heart diseases induce central breathing disturbances. CSR is a marker of poor prognosis in patients with heart failure (HF).[6] On the other hand, optimal treatment of CSR significantly improves the survival of such patients.[7] Based on these findings, it is reasonable to screen HF patients systematically for SRBD, even if they do not suffer from daytime sleepiness or witnessed apneas. Because of the unfavorable consequences, specific treatment of CSR should be

a Institute of Pneumology, University Witten/Herdecke, Clinic for Pneumology and Allergology, Center of Sleep Medicine and Respiratory Care, Bethanien Hospital, Aufderhöherstraße 169-175, Solingen 42699, Germany; b College of Medicine, University of Cincinnati, Sleepcare Diagnostics, Mason, OH, USA
* Corresponding author.
E-mail address: randerath@klinik-bethanien.de

Sleep Med Clin 9 (2014) 69–85
http://dx.doi.org/10.1016/j.jsmc.2013.11.001
1556-407X/14/$ – see front matter © 2014 Elsevier Inc. All rights reserved.

applied as soon as possible if breathing disorders still remain after optimizing cardiac medication and interventional therapy.[8]

Unfortunately, several therapeutic approaches have failed to sufficiently reduce CSR and other central breathing disturbances. There are conflicting results on the supplementation of oxygen during the night and on treatment with the carbonic anhydrase inhibitor acetazolamide.[9–13] Oxygen may reduce the apnea-hypopnea index (AHI; defined as the number of apneas and hypopneas per hour of sleep) by about 14 to 18 per hour in absolute figures in CSR.[14] However, this means only a 50% reduction in comparison with baseline, which is similar to the effect of CPAP. Oxygen improved the left ventricular ejection fraction (LVEF) in 1 of 3 studies.[14] Based on these limited data, the American Academy of Sleep Medicine has concluded that a trial may be reasonable.[14]

CPAP has demonstrated improvement in LVEF and survival in HF patients who suffer from CSR.[5,15] Although CPAP reduces the AHI by less than 50% according to several short-term and long-term studies,[16,17] it improves the increased work of breathing, the ventilation-perfusion relationship in the lungs, the oxygen demand and oxygen supply, and the left ventricular afterload and the cardiac index in HF patients.[5,15,18–28] Despite these encouraging findings, the CANPAP trial failed to confirm a benefit in survival under CPAP treatment.[16] However, a post hoc analysis of the study showed an improved survival in those patients whose SRBD were sufficiently reduced when compared with those with insufficient change. There are very limited data on the treatment of CSR using bilevel positive airway pressure (BPAP). Because of the small body of evidence BPAP should only be considered in individual cases.[14]

The most important conclusion from these data is that the prognosis of CSR patients essentially depends on the optimal suppression of SRBDs.[7] CPAP and BPAP mechanically influence preload and afterload of the heart, but this does not suffice. The fixed pressure support does not allow for counterbalancing the waxing and waning of the flow amplitude. Therefore, an approach more precisely addressing the complex pathophysiology would seem to be crucial in overcoming CSR and CSA and achieving optimal outcome.

PATHOPHYSIOLOGIC BACKGROUND

CSR is typically characterized by an alternation of apneas and/or hypopneas and prolonged hyperventilation in a crescendo-decrescendo pattern of the tidal volume.[2] Respiratory drive and consecutively breathing effort are reduced during central apneas. However, the hyperpneic periods are longer, and the increase and decrease of the ventilation less abrupt, in CSR in comparison with other forms of CSA. Thus, elevation and diminishment of ventilatory drive and consecutively ventilatory effort coexist in CSR. As a result, CSR is characterized by a net hyperventilation with reduced $Paco_2$. The pathophysiology includes several mosaic pieces leading to a vicious circle:

- Fluid overload in the lungs of HF patients stimulates vagal afferents, which increase breathing frequency.
- The reduction of cardiac output slows the blood flow to the chemoreceptors, leading to delayed reactions to changes of the CO_2.
- Hypersensitivity of peripheral and central chemoreceptors leads to overshooting or undershooting of the ventilation, and the hypoxic and hypercapnic ventilatory response is elevated.

As a result, respiration becomes unstable and the typical pattern of waxing and waning of the flow amplitude appears.[8]

ADAPTIVE SERVOVENTILATION
Devices and Algorithms

Adaptive servoventilation (ASV) has been developed to counterbalance the continuous shift between hyperventilation and hypoventilation and, therefore, to more effectively improve CSA/CSR. Moreover, ASV may also normalize the elevated apneic threshold that substantially contributes to the pathophysiology of CSR and CSA.

Three devices have been released that analyze the patient's breathing pattern (flow or minute ventilation) in a moving average throughout the night and modulate the pressure support anticyclically. If a predefined limit of the target parameter is not reached, additional pressure support is supplied. If the limit is overcome, pressure support is reduced. The algorithms are called Adaptive Servo-Ventilation (Resmed, Bella Vista, Australia), Auto Servo-Ventilation (Philips Respironics, Murrysville, PA, USA), and Anticyclic Modulated Ventilation (Weinmann, Hamburg, Germany). However, the term ASV is often used to generally describe the principle of treatment.

The devices commonly apply 2 pressure levels. The expiratory positive airway pressure (EPAP) serves to sustain upper airway patency. The difference between the actual inspiratory positive airway pressure (IPAP) and the expiratory pressure defines the pressure support, which is essential to overcome central hypopneas and CSR when required (**Fig. 1**).[8] Whereas BPAP devices apply

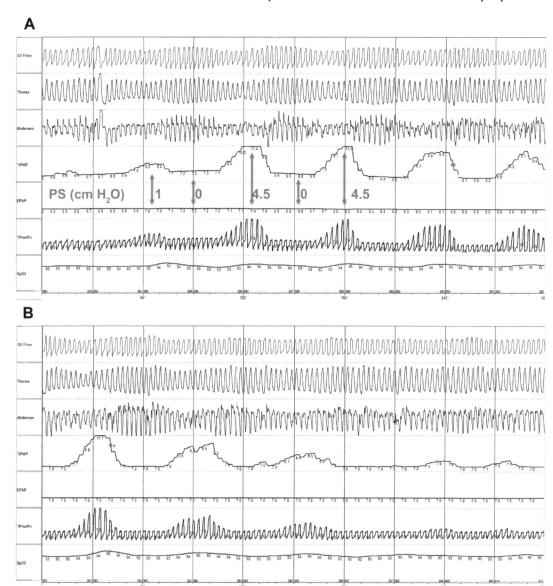

Fig. 1. The reaction of ASV devices to variations in tidal volume. (*A*) An example of Cheyne-Stokes respiration with waxing and waning of flow and effort. During periods of hypoventilation the difference between IPAP and EPAP increases, whereas it is reduced during periods of hyperventilation. The pressure support (PS, *light blue numbers*) varies between 0 and 4.5 cm H_2O. Device: BiPAP auto SV advanced; 5 minutes. (*B, C*) Later periods from the same patient during the same night. The respiratory pattern has almost normalized. However, the underlying Cheyne-Stokes respiration is recognized from the ranges in pressure support. Device: BiPAP auto SV advanced; 5 minutes. (*D*) Ten-minute period of Cheyne-Stokes respiration with continued increase of inspiratory pressure and pressure support. As there are no obstructive disturbances, the EPAP is not varied. During the second half of the period the pressure support is reduced, as it is not needed because of hyperventilation. Device: BiPAP Auto SV advanced. (*E*) The reaction of the algorithm in more detail. The red line shows the variations of the peak inspiratory pressure, the dark blue line the variation of the lowest EPAP, and the light blue line the end-expiratory pressure. During periods with high minute ventilation (*left part of the figure*) the difference between IPAP and EPAP (the pressure support) is low. When the minute ventilation decreases (*middle part of the figure*), the difference between IPAP and EPAP (the pressure support) increases, by both elevating IPAP and reducing EPAP. The end-expiratory pressure remains stable, as there is no evidence of obstructive disturbances. Device: SomnoVent CR; 1 minute. Abdomen, effort channel—abdomen; Druck, pressure; EPAP, expiratory positive airway pressure; In/Ex, indication of inspiration and expiration as measured by the device; IPAP, inspiratory positive airway pressure; Lage, body position; PresPn, pressure measured by the device; Puls, pulse; rel. AMV, relative minute ventilation; Resp. Flow, respiratory flow as measured by the device; Schnarchen, snoring; SpO2, oxygen saturation; SV Flow, respiratory flow as measured by the device; Thorax, effort channel—thorax.

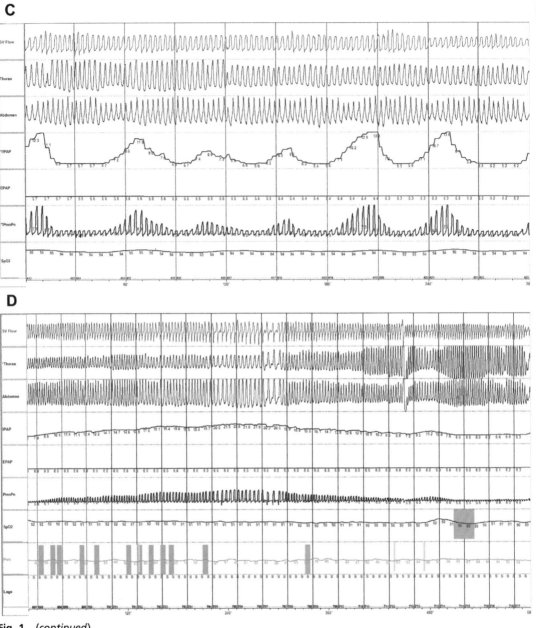

Fig. 1. (*continued*)

one predefined difference between inspiration and expiration and therefore deliver one fixed tidal volume, under ASV it changes continuously. In cases of central apnea the ASV devices apply mandatory breaths (**Fig. 2**). The physician can choose between a manually fixed and an automatic backup frequency. The most recent versions of the algorithms combine both automatic CPAP and ASV (**Fig. 3**).

The ASV devices differ in terms of the target parameter (flow or minute ventilation), backup frequency, pressure ranges, and minimal pressure support that can be applied (Javaheri et al, in preparation, 2014). ResMed (AutoSet CS, VPAP Adapt, VPAP Adapt Enhanced, S9 VPAP Adapt) released the first ASV algorithm, which compared the actual minute ventilation with a target on the basis of a 3-minute moving average. If the actual ventilation is lower than 90% of the average, the device increases the pressure support. The first versions of the algorithm delivered a minimum pressure support of 3 mbar and were not capable

E

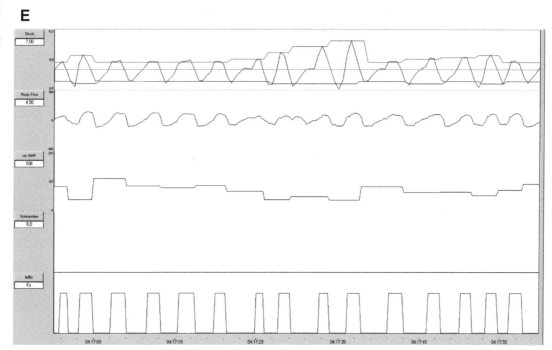

Fig. 1. (*continued*)

of working in CPAP mode in periods of pure obstructive disturbances. The user had to predefine the end-expiratory pressure (EEP) between 4 and 10 mbar and the minimum (3–6 mbar plus EEP) and maximum (8–15 mbar plus EEP) pressure support. The backup frequency was set automatically. However, the actual model of the device can work not only in ASV mode but also in ASV with automatic adaptation of EEP, or in CPAP mode. For the ASV modes the clinician has to define a minimal and maximal pressure support. In addition, the physician fixes EPAP in the ASV mode while a pressure range is defined for the EPAP in ASV with automatic EPAP.

By contrast, the Respironics algorithm (BiPAP AutoSV, BiPAP AutoSV Advanced) focuses on the peak flow as a target parameter, which is compared with a 4-minute moving average (Javaheri et al, in preparation, 2014). Expiratory and minimum inspiratory pressure can be set on the same level, allowing the device to run in CPAP mode if there is no need for pressure support. In the first versions of the device, the investigator had to determine the EPAP to sustain upper airway patency between 4 and 25 mbar (based on a previous manual CPAP titration), the minimum (IPAP-min) and maximum IPAP (IPAPmax), both being between 4 and 30 mbar. The actual IPAP varies between IPAPmin and IPAPmax to maintain a target inspiratory airflow and therefore to eliminate

CSA/CSR events. The device provides an automatic backup rate. However, the user is able to fix the backup frequency manually between 4/min and 30/min. The most recent versions (BiPAP Auto SV Advanced) determine the EPAP automatically within a range that must be defined by the clinician. Pressure support is automatically varied between 0 and 20 cm H_2O above the prevailing EPAP.

The SOMNOventCR (Weinmann, Hamburg, Germany) was the first device to combine automatic CPAP and ASV (Javaheri et al, in preparation, 2014). The anticyclic modulated ventilation (ACMV) algorithm is regulated based on flow, pressure, and snoring signals. The minute ventilation is compared with the previous average minute ventilation in a moving window and is focused mainly (but not only) on the last 2 minutes. The device applies 3 pressure levels: the IPAP, the expiratory pressure in the early expiration (EPAP), and the end-expiratory positive airway pressure (EEPAP). The investigator has to determine 2 pressure levels: the minimum EEPAP and the maximum IPAP. In the case of upper airway obstructions, such as obstructive apneas or hypopneas, flow limitations, or snoring, the device increases the EEPAP automatically. During CSR the difference between IPAP and EPAP is continuously increased to raise the tidal volume. During hyperventilation the difference can reach CPAP

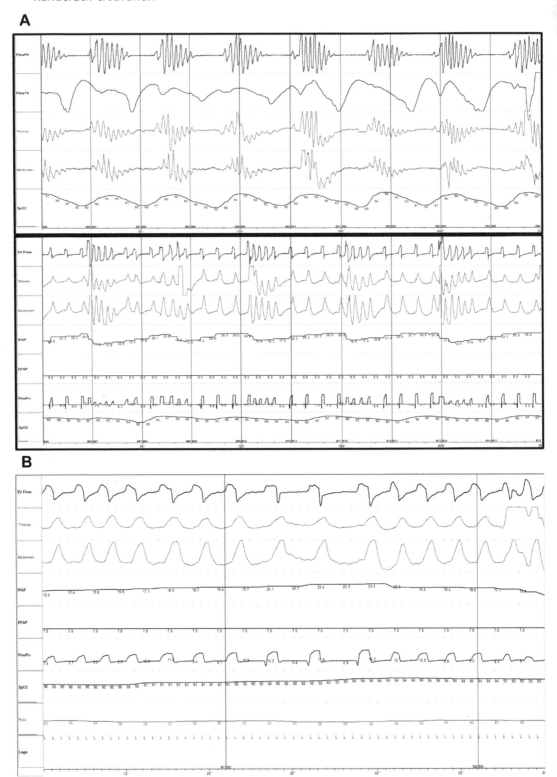

Fig. 2. Mandatory breaths in central apneas. (*A*) The upper part shows the typical pattern of Cheyne-Stokes respiration with waxing and waning of flow and effort and consecutive oxygen desaturations. The lower part shows mandatory breaths during central apneas. Note the regular application of mandatory breaths. The peak pressure of these breaths increases step by step with respiratory pressure. (*B*) Central apneas treated with 3 consecutive mandatory breaths (*middle part of the figure*). The pressure support of these breaths increases step by step. Device: BiPAP Auto SV advanced; 1 minute/page. FlowP4, oral nasal flow; FlowTh, thorax flow. Other abbreviations: see **Fig. 1**.

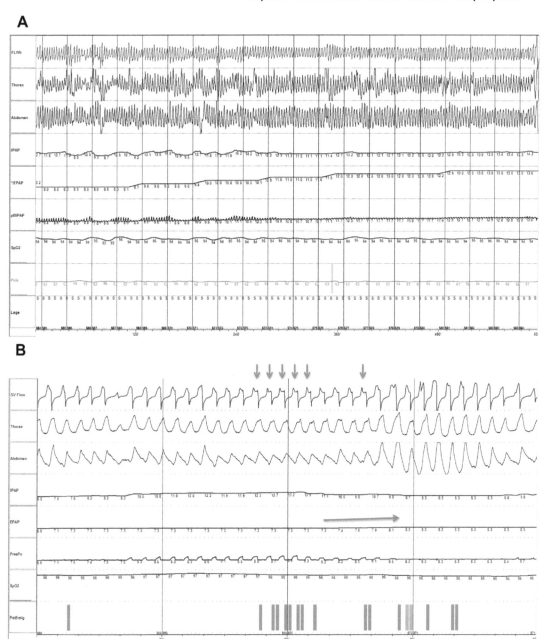

Fig. 3. The reaction during obstructive events. The advanced ASV devices counterbalance upper airway obstruction by increasing expiratory pressures. (*A*) A 10-minute period in a patient with coexisting Cheyne-Stokes respiration and obstructive sleep apnea. The EPAP increases (*left half of the figure*) because of obstructive hypopneas. Device: BiPAP Auto SV advanced. (*B, C*) The reaction of the algorithm in more detail (2 minutes). The device detects a reduction of flow and increases the IPAP slightly as a consequence. As there is no sufficient improvement, the device consecutively increases the EPAP. The flow channel indicates flattening as a clear marker of upper airway obstruction. Device: BiPAP Auto SV advanced. (*D*) The pressure (derived from the mask) varies during inspiration and expiration. EPAP increases on the right part of the figure. The IPAP increases consecutively to maintain pressure support on the previous level. However, at the end the difference between EPAP and IPAP increases according to hypoventilation. Device: SomnoVent CR; 10 minutes. (*E*) Detailed presentation of the variation of early expiratory pressure and end-expiratory pressure. The pressure support (difference between IPAP and EPAP) varies according to reductions of minute ventilation in a first attempt. The end-EPAP (*light blue line*) is elevated if increases of pressure support fail to improve minute ventilation or if there are additional parameters of upper airway obstruction (flattening, snoring). FLW6: Flow measured at the mask. Druck Maske, pressure measured by the mask; Flow Gerät, respiratory flow as measured by the device; PatEreig, patient events; pBIPAP, bilevel pressure as measured by the device. Other abbreviations: see **Fig. 1**.

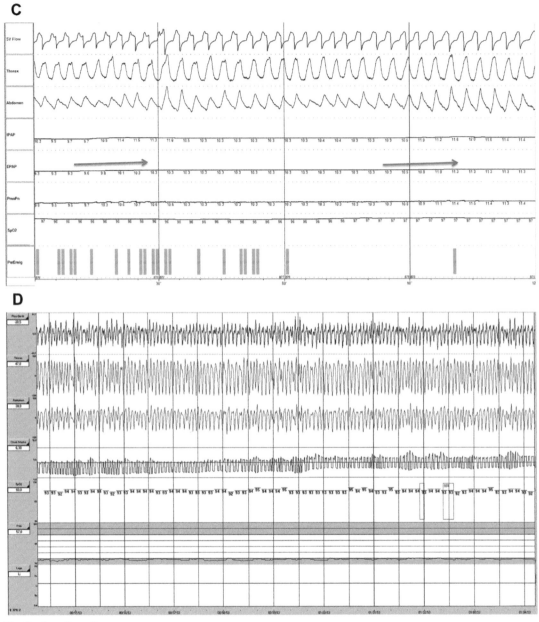

Fig. 3. (continued)

level. Mandatory breaths are applied automatically with a frequency depending on the patient's baseline respiratory rate.

Titration and Setting of ASV

In clinical practice, the setting of maximum inspiratory pressure under ASV depends on suspected cardiovascular side effects. For testing, it is advisable to apply the maximum inspiratory pressure during wakefulness and control the arterial blood pressure in patients with severe or unstable HF.

If the expiratory pressure is not determined automatically, it can also be defined based on manual titration. Hence, a CPAP trial is reasonable for 2 reasons: (1) it allows the definition of the expiratory pressure level needed to overcome obstructive events, and (2) if CPAP efficiently normalizes respiration, ASV can be avoided. The minimal pressure support for home treatment can be set based on the findings of an in-hospital ASV trial using the largest possible inspiratory range. If the actually applied IPAP during this trial is on the lowest level for large time periods, the

E

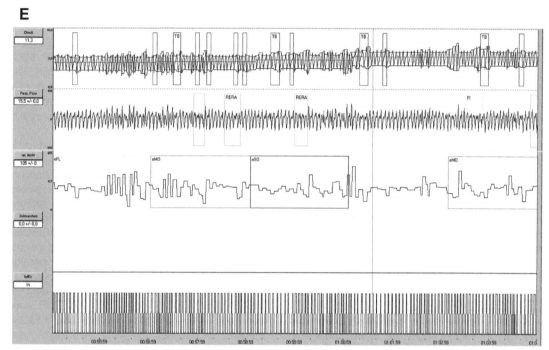

Fig. 3. (*continued*)

IPAPmin can be set to 0 cm H_2O. Otherwise, if the patient continuously needs higher pressure support during the trial, it might be advantageous to predefine an additional support to stabilize breathing.[8]

Influence of ASV on Respiratory Disturbances and Cardiovascular Parameters

The efficacy of ASV in the treatment of CSR has been studied intensively in case series and follow-up studies, but also in short-term and long-term randomized controlled trials. Teschler and colleagues[17] compared ASV (AutoSet CS) with oxygen, BPAP, and CPAP in a randomized order for 1 night each in 14 stable HF patients under optimal medical treatment (New York Heart Association [NYHA] functional class II–III, fractional shortening 0.19). The patients had predominantly CSA/CSR with fewer than 10 obstructive disturbances per hour. The investigators demonstrated significant improvements in the central respiratory disturbances during sleep under ASV therapy. As in the CANPAP trial, they found a reduction of the AHI by half under CPAP while ASV improved SRBDs by greater than 80%. The effect of CPAP was similar to that of oxygen, which confirmed previous findings.[17,29]

There are no studies comparing the different ASV devices. However, the efficacy of ASV in comparison with CPAP, BPAP, or standard therapy has been confirmed with all devices. For example, Arzt and colleagues[30] studied 14 patients suffering of chronic HF (ejection fraction [EF]<45%) and a portion of CSA/CSR of more than 80% at inclusion. The patients were enrolled for treatment with ASV (BiPAP AutoSV) after being insufficiently treated with CPAP or BPAP over a period of 27 ± 11 weeks. CPAP or BPAP significantly reduced the AHI by half compared with the diagnostic evaluation, as has been shown previously. By contrast, ASV normalized all respiratory parameters.

Promising preliminary data were found on the combination treatment of automatic positive airway pressure (PAP) and ASV. In a pilot trial of treatment over 2 weeks (Vent CR, ACMV), 12 patients with coexisting OSAS and CSR/CSA were studied. Seven suffered from arterial hypertension, coronary heart disease, and mitral regurgitation, and none of congestive HF. The algorithm normalized all types of coexisting OSA and CSA/CSR, and improved the sleep profile and arousal figures.[31]

Javaheri and colleagues[32] conducted a randomized controlled trial in patients from 5 sleep centers, which compared CPAP and the two different modes of ASV (BiPAP AutoSV), one fixed and one with automatic adjustment of EPAP. Whereas CPAP reduced the mean AHI from 53 ± 23 to 35 ± 20 events/h, the ASV algorithms suppressed respiratory disturbances to 10 ± 10 events/h (conventional ASV) and 6 ± 6/h (advanced ASV). Both ASV algorithms were equally effective in the resolution of OSA when compared with CPAP. Once again, the data support previous findings that CPAP reduces the total AHI in CSA by approximately 50%, and that ASV is superior to CPAP in the suppression of hypopneas as well as central and mixed apneas. Of note, the advanced ASV device conferred an additional improvement in central disturbances in comparison with conventional BiPAP AutoSV.[32,33]

ASV actually interferes with the pathophysiology of CSR. CPAP may influence SRBD in several ways: it stabilizes the upper airways and counterbalances upper airway obstruction; the positive thoracic pressure reduces left ventricular afterload and therefore improves LVEF; and CPAP can enlarge lung volumes and reduce ventilation-perfusion mismatch. However, CPAP does not substantially influence breathing rhythm and chemosensitivity. Conventional BPAP applies a fixed pressure support even in situations of the patient's hyperventilation, which might aggravate hypocapnia and propagate overshooting and undershooting of ventilation. By contrast, ASV combines the effects of CPAP with variable pressure support and the application of mandatory breaths. Therefore, disturbances of respiratory drive and periods of hypoventilation or hyperventilation can be counterbalanced. Sufficient pressure support during hypoventilation normalizes oxygen saturation and prevents hypoxic ventilatory response. Regarding ASV, Oldenburg and colleagues[34] followed 105 patients with chronic HF with an EF less than 40% and CSR for a mean of 6.7 months. Patients who rejected ASV therapy, or used it on less than 50% of the nights or fewer than 4 hours per day were compares with those who adhered sufficiently to the therapy. ASV significantly improved CSR, HF class, LVEF, oxygen uptake, and 6-minute walk distance. The investigators also studied hypercapnic ventilatory response, which was significantly reduced by sufficient ASV use. Thus ASV reduces the increased chemosensitivity of CSR patients.

Several studies included primarily patients with almost pure CSR/CSA. However, in clinical practice patients with pure CSA are rarely found. Furthermore, many patients with OSAS show at least a minor proportion of central disturbances, and PAP may induce CSA/CSR in a small percentage of patients (CPAP-emerging CSA).[35,36] Therefore, the authors performed a prospective, observational pilot study on the efficacy of ASV (BiPAP AutoSV) was performed in 10 consecutive male patients with coexisting OSAS and CSA/CSR with and without HF over 8 weeks. ASV proved to effectively suppress all types of SRBD,

and improved sleep quality. The results were similar between patients with and without cardiovascular disease.[37] Kasai and colleagues[38] confirmed these findings in 31 HF patients (EF<50%, NYHA II–IV) with coexisting OSA and CSR who were randomized to receive either CPAP or ASV for 3 months. ASV more effectively suppressed respiratory disturbances, and improved the quality of life and LVEF.

Most recently, a randomized controlled study in patients with coexisting OSA and CSA in mild to moderate HF was performed. Seventy patients with arterial hypertension, coronary heart disease, or cardiomyopathy were treated for 12 months with CPAP or ASV. ASV was equally effective as CPAP in suppressing obstructive disturbances, but was significantly superior regarding central events. In addition, brain natriuretic peptide (BNP) as a marker of cardiac function was significantly more improved with ASV.[39] The data on the efficacy of ASV on SRBD and BNP have been confirmed by Arzt and colleagues.[40] Stable chronic HF patients (EF≤40%, AHI≥20/h) were randomized to ASV to optimal cardiologic management with or without ASV. The investigators demonstrated a significant reduction of respiratory disturbances and BNP under ASV. Despite the improvements of cardiac markers, these studies[39,40] did not demonstrate increases of LVEF, which may be due to the population (mild HF) or the design (duration).[39,40]

However, several randomized and nonrandomized studies showed improvements in left ventricular function.[14,38,41–43] Yoshihisa and colleagues[44] performed a nonrandomized cohort study in 60 patients with stable congestive HF and CSR (NYHA II–IV, LVEF 38.7%, AHI 36.8/h). Twenty-three patients agreed to use ASV while 37 refused this option. Along with the normalization of respiratory disturbances, oxygen saturation, and sleep parameters, ASV improved cardiac outcome (NYHA functional class, echocardiographic parameters, and BNP) in comparison with baseline and non-ASV over 6 months. Of importance, there was a significant reduction of cardiovascular deaths or rehospitalizations from HF under ASV.

Using a similar design, Koyama and colleagues[45] investigated the influence of ASV on renal function in 27 HF patients treated with ASV in a comparison with 16 without ASV over 12 months. Active treatment significantly improved glomerular filtration rate, LVEF, and high-sensitivity C-reactive protein (CRP). The increase of renal function correlated with the improvement in LVEF and the inflammatory marker.

Cardiac resynchronization therapy (CRT) and biventricular pacing has become an important part of

HF treatment because it leads to substantial improvement in heart function, quality of life, and survival. Miyata and colleagues[46] studied the question of whether ASV therapy might additionally improve the outcome of HF patients with CSR. Therefore, they randomized 22 patients after CRT defibrillator implantation to standard therapy or additional ASV. While both groups showed improvement of LVEF, the investigators found a significant difference in improvement of the BNP level and in the proportion of event-free patients in the ASV group.

Influence of ASV on Physiologic Parameters and Sympathoadrenergic Activity

There have been concerns that the application of PAP in CSR might negatively influence hemodynamics immediately. Thus, Yamada and colleagues[47] performed right heart catheterization in 34 patients with chronic stable HF and 11 controls during wakefulness without breathing disturbances, so that the mechanical influences of PAP on the heart were separated from the influences on SRBD and oxygen supply. ASV significantly reduced the stroke volume index (SVI) in healthy controls but not in HF patients. SVI improved under ASV in those HF patients with high pulmonary capillary wedge pressure and mitral regurgitation. Therefore, the study is consistent with previous findings on the application of CPAP or BPAP, which decrease cardiac output in normal persons owing to reduction of the venous return. However, PAP application improves cardiac function in HF acutely by reducing preload, thus improving functional mitral regurgitation and the morphology of the heart.[48–50]

Haruki and colleagues[51] compared the influence of ASV on echocardiographic parameters in 15 patients treated with ASV and 11 who refused the therapy. The study included a short-term trial (30 minutes) and a 24-week follow-up period. During the acute trial, ASV reduced heart rate and systolic and diastolic blood pressure, and increased stroke volume and cardiac output. These changes were associated with increases in systemic arterial compliance and vascular resistance, indicating the role of an improvement in the left ventricular afterload under ASV therapy. In addition, active treatment improved NYHA class and cardiac function over the 24-week follow-up period, whereas there were no significant changes in the control group.

Increased sympathetic activity is a marker of pour outcome. Therefore, Harada and colleagues[52] asked whether ASV influences sympathetic activity in HF with or without CSR. The investigators measured muscle sympathetic nerve activity (MSNA) in addition to cardiac and respiratory parameters, including the variation of tidal volume as a marker of respiratory instability. The 11 patients with periodic breathing showed a modest positive correlation between MSNA and respiratory instability, which was not found in the 18 patients without periodic breathing. ASV reduced respiratory parameters and, consecutively, MSNA. It was concluded that ASV reduced MSNA by slowing the respiratory rate and stabilizing the breathing pattern. In addition, Pepperell and colleagues[53] showed a reduction of catecholamines under effective ASV therapy in a randomized controlled trial.

Efficacy According to Severity of SRBD or Underlying Cardiac Disease

For clinicians, it is most relevant to know which patients should be treated with ASV. As many patients do not suffer from clinical symptoms, such as daytime sleepiness, treatment is often initiated based on the severity of SRBD. Different thresholds of the AHI between 5/h and 30/h are recommended. Takama and Kurabayashi[54] asked whether the efficacy of ASV differs according to the severity of SRBD in HF patients with NYHA class II–IV. Sixty-one patients were divided into 3 groups according to the AHI (<20/h, 20–40/h, >40/h). There were no significant differences between the groups in terms of anthropometric parameters, underlying cardiac disease, severity of HF, and drug therapy. After 6 months of treatment, OSA, CSA/CSR, and BNP improved significantly in all groups. Moreover, LVEF increased in all subgroups but failed to reach statistical significance in mild sleep apnea. These findings were confirmed by Koyama and colleagues,[55] who followed 38 HF patients for 1 year and compared compliant with noncompliant patients. The investigators found a significant reduction of survival and lower LVEF in noncompliant patients in both moderate to severe SRBD (AHI≥20/h) and mild SRBD (AHI<20/h). These findings, albeit from cohort studies, support that ASV might be beneficial independent of the severity of SRDB.

As mentioned earlier, patients with HF and SRBD suffer from less daytime sleepiness in comparison with the general population or patients with SRBD without HF.[56] However, treatment compliance depends crucially on the awareness of the symptoms and their improvement under treatment.[57] Thus, HF patients with SRBD are at risk of noncompliance. Koyama and colleagues[58] addressed whether limited ASV usage is associated with cardiovascular improvement. A group of 86 HF patients was retrospectively divided into 3 groups according to their compliance. After

6 months, those patients who used their devices for longer than 4 h/d or 1 to 4 h/d showed a significant improvement of LVEF and BNP in comparison with those who used their devices for less than 1 h/d. In addition, the increase in LVEF and the decrease in BNP correlated significantly with the daily use of ASV. Therefore, patients should be encouraged to use their devices for more than 4 hours. However, even limited use might improve cardiac function.

Most studies in HF with CSR included patients with an EF of less than 40%, which is typical for systolic left ventricular failure. However, diastolic HF is also associated with increased prevalence of CSR. Diastolic HF leads to pulmonary congestion and stimulation of intrapulmonary vagal irritant receptors, and therefore predisposes to respiratory instability. Bitter and colleagues[59] followed 60 patients with diastolic HF and CSR for 1 year, 39 of whom accepted ASV and 21 of whom refused treatment or used it insufficiently. ASV led to significant improvement of SRBD, oxygen saturation, and parameters of cardiopulmonary exercise testing and echocardiography.

Does ASV Influence Daytime Symptoms and Quality of Life?

Pepperell and colleagues[53] performed a randomized, controlled, double-blind study comparing effective (AutoSet CS) with subtherapeutic ASV over 1 month (pressure 1.75 cm H_2O, pressure support 0.75–2.75 cm H_2O, 30 HF patients of NYHA II–IV, LVEF 33%–36%). The investigators focused primarily on parameters regarding sleep quality and daytime performance, and found a significant improvement in excessive daytime sleepiness, BNP, and metadrenaline excretion under therapeutic ASV.

In addition, Philippe and colleagues[43] studied efficacy and compliance under ASV in comparison with CPAP. Twenty-five patients with CSA/CSR and stable HF (NYHA II–IV) were randomly assigned to receive 1 of the 2 treatment options for 6 months. ASV proved to be superior to CPAP in terms of AHI, LVEF, and compliance. Whereas the daily use of CPAP decreased under CPAP, it improved under ASV at 6 months. There were no significant improvements in daytime sleepiness (Epworth Sleepiness Scale). However, the scores were low at baseline, which is common in CSR. Therefore there was only limited room for improvement. Nevertheless, compared with CPAP the quality of life measured with the Minnesota Questionnaire improved significantly with ASV.

Alternatives to ASV

The application of oxygen might interfere with the pathophysiology of CSR or CSA by improving oxygen supply to the heart, brain, and respiratory muscles, or by reducing hypoxic ventilatory response. Yoshihisa and colleagues[60] addressed whether ASV or oxygen influence the pathophysiology of heart function and markers of progression and prognosis of HF. These investigators compared ASV and oxygen in 42 HF patients (EF 34.6%, predominant CSA) for 1 night. Both options, oxygen and ASV, normalized the oxygen desaturation index and the arousal index. However, whereas oxygen reduced the AHI by only 50%, AHI was normalized under ASV. In addition, ASV was superior in terms of parameters of cardiac overload (arterial natriuretic peptide, BNP) and sympathetic nervous activity (plasma noradrenaline, urinary catecholamines). No difference was found in parameters of inflammation and cardiac damage between oxygen and ASV (troponin T, high-sensitivity CRP). These data indicate that correction of oxygenation alone does not suffice to improve HF. Normalization of respiratory disturbances and mechanical influences on the heart seem to play a crucial role in sufficient treatment of HF with SRBD.

As mentioned earlier, the prevailing $Paco_2$ and its relation to the apnea threshold substantially influence CSR. By counterbalancing overshooting and undershooting of ventilation, ASV normalizes hypocapnia and hypercapnia. Similarly, the application of CO_2 or the enlargement of dead space can increase the actual $Paco_2$ and thus reduce CSA. Szollosi and colleagues[61] compared the influence of dead space and ASV in 10 male HF patients with CSA in a randomized crossover design. Both reduced respiratory disturbances similarly and significantly in comparison with a control night without therapy. However, dead space was associated with an impairment of sleep quality (increased arousal index and reduction of total sleep time).

Open Questions on ASV Therapy in HF Patients with SRBD

Summarizing these results, ASV has proved to be highly effective in improving CSR. This method is superior to other positive pressure approaches, such as CPAP, BPAP, or noninvasive ventilation. Although several studies were performed in small groups and nonrandomized designs (treatment follow-up), there is growing evidence from randomized controlled trials. Nevertheless, sufficient prospective data on survival and severe cardiac events over the longer term are urgently needed.

These questions are addressed in the 2 large international, multicenter, randomized controlled studies (SERVE-HF, ADVENT-HF) on cardiovascular outcome and long-term efficacy.[62]

Besides the consistent findings on the suppression of all phenotypes of SRBD under ASV, the observation of treatment failure in single patients should be carefully considered. From the authors' point of view, most importantly mask leakages may lead to treatment failure as shown by Pusalavidyasagar and colleagues.[63] Active or passive closure of the upper airways (closed central apneas)[64] seems to be another rare cause for insufficient treatment of CSR with ASV. This phenomenon can be supposed if an increase of the tidal volume does not normalize CSR. The complexity of the problem and the comorbidity indicate that close supervision and optimal management of the interface in the sleep laboratory is crucial in patients treated with technologically advanced devices.[8] Although the advanced devices allow for automatic titration of EPAP and pressure support, precise settings of the predefined pressure range and close supervision of the patient during the initiation night remains the duty of the sleep specialist, as pointed out by Javaheri and colleagues.[32] The advantage of autoadjusting devices, especially in complicated breathing patterns, is not a cost reduction by saving labor but a more precise adaptation of the pressures according to their sophisticated algorithms.

ASV IN COMPLEX SLEEP APNEA AND OTHER CENTRAL DISTURBANCES

There are no prospective controlled trials on ASV in idiopathic CSA, high-altitude CSA, or other forms of central disturbances. Kuzniar and colleagues[65] retrospectively analyzed the efficacy of different therapeutic approaches in their patients with CSA, but did not only include patients with pure CSA. These investigators found that ASV was superior to oxygen, CPAP, and bilevel therapy. The same group compared ASV and noninvasive positive pressure ventilation (NPPV) in patients with CSA/CSR, complex sleep apnea, and mixed sleep apnea. Both options sufficiently improved respiratory disturbances while ASV was more effective than NPPV.[66]

Allam and colleagues[67] presented retrospective data from 100 patients with CPAP-emerging CSA (complex sleep apnea), pure CSA in cardiac diseases, chronic obstructive pulmonary disease, cerebrovascular diseases, and chronic opioid intake, and in CSR/CSA. All patients had undergone a CPAP trial that had failed, and were thereafter treated with BPAP in spontaneous mode (BPAP-S), BPAP in spontaneous-timed mode (BPAP-ST), CPAP or BPAP with oxygen, and ASV. Whereas BPAP-S led to an insignificant increase, the other options improved SRBD. However, ASV was clearly superior to the other therapies in all patient groups.

Carnevale and colleagues[68] retrospectively analyzed data from 74 patients who suffered from HF-induced and non–HF-induced hypocapnic central disturbances and were treated with ASV. The analysis included 41 patients with underlying neurologic diseases or idiopathic CSA, and 33 cardiac patients. The HF patients were older (60 ± 14 vs 69 ± 11 years, $P<.002$) and less sleepy compared with the non-HF patients (Epworth Sleepiness Scale 10.7 ± 5.3 vs 6.8 ± 4.7, $P<.002$). The mean follow-up was 36 ± 18 months. The overall compliance was 5.9 ± 2.9 h/night (non-HF patients) versus 5.2 ± 2.6 h/night (HF patients). ASV significantly improved breathing disturbances, oxygen saturation, and $Paco_2$. Moreover, it improved daytime sleepiness and EF in compliant patients.[68]

These studies are limited by the nonrandomized, partly retrospective design and the heterogeneous populations, so that they do not allow for final conclusions but for generation of hypotheses. The data have yet to be confirmed in well-designed prospective studies in clearly defined patient groups.

ASV IN OPIOID-INDUCED SLEEP APNEA

Opioids are increasingly prescribed not only to relieve pain but also, for example, to alleviate dyspnea in patients with chronic pulmonary disorders. In addition, opiate addiction remains an unsolved problem, with an increasing number of patients abusing opioids or being treated in methadone maintenance programs.[69] These epidemiologic findings are associated with observations of SRBD, including perioperative complications in children and adults.[70] In 2007, Walker and colleagues[71] described different phenotypes of SRBD under opioids (obstructive disturbances, central apneas, ataxic or irregular respiration, sustained hypoventilation).

The pathophysiology of opioid-induced sleep apnea (OISA) differs substantially from that of hyperventilatory central disturbances, such as CSR. Pattinson[72] described shallow and irregular respiration leading to hypercapnia and hypoxia. Opioids inhibit the respiratory rhythms by suppressing brainstem activity, leading to reduced breathing frequency. Peripheral and central chemosensitivity play a major pathophysiologic role, leading to a diminishment of the hypoxic and hypercapnic ventilatory response. Moreover, opioids impede the activity of the upper airway muscles, which predisposes to obstructive disturbances. Therefore, in essence OISA represents a hypercapnic phenotype of sleep apnea.

Because of the complex pathophysiology, optimal therapy is still under discussion. In 2008, 2 studies with contradictory results were published in the same issue of the *Journal of Clinical Sleep Medicine*. Whereas Farney and colleagues[73] failed to show a difference between CPAP and ASV, Javaheri and colleagues[74] found an effective treatment with ASV in a small group of patients with opioid-induced sleep apnea. However, more recently Ramar and colleagues[75] investigated retrospectively CPAP nonresponders with central breathing disturbances caused by chronic HF or use of opioids, and found that ASV enabled sufficient therapy in most patients in both groups. Although this was not a randomized CPAP or placebo-controlled trial, the investigators analyzed the largest sample to date in a real-life situation. Future studies should address the question as to why 30% to 40% of patients with HF and OISA, respectively, could not be treated optimally.

SUMMARY

The number of patients suffering from CSA/CSR or coexisting OSAS and CSA/CSR presenting in sleep clinics is rapidly increasing, owing to the growing population of the elderly in Western societies, the increasing incidence of cardiovascular comorbidities, the advancements in cardiologic treatment options, and the higher awareness of the problem in the medical community. Although data on survival are still missing, ASV has proved to be superior to CPAP, BPAP, and noninvasive ventilation in terms of SRBD in patients with or without HF. Based on pathophysiologic considerations and clinical results, the authors try to optimize any underlying disease, especially cardiovascular or cerebrovascular disorders, renal failure, or chronic opioid use in patients with central SRBD. If breathing disturbances remain a short-term CPAP trial is conducted, which is supported by a 50% response rate and improvements of LVEF. However, data on BPAP therapy or oxygen supply do not encourage the authors to generally use these approaches. Therefore, a switch to ASV is made if CPAP fails. There is consistent evidence demonstrating that ASV normalizes the different phenotypes of SRBD and is higher effective in terms of CSA/CSR, in comparison with CPAP. In addition, short-term and long-term data indicate that ASV improves cardiac parameters and quality of life, and interferes with the underlying pathophysiology of CSA/CSR. However, clinicians have yet to elucidate the reasons for ineffective treatment in a portion of patients. Moreover, as yet it remains unknown whether improvements in SRBD, cardiac measures, and surrogate parameters translate into a better long-term outcome with regard to overall survival and exercise performance.

REFERENCES

1. Sullivan CE, Issa FG, Berthon-Jones M, et al. Reversal of obstructive sleep apnoea by continuous positive airway pressure applied through the nares. Lancet 1981;1:862–5.
2. American Academy of Sleep Medicine. International classification of sleep disorders. Diagnostic and coding manual. 2nd edition. Westchester (IL): American Academy of Sleep Medicine; 2005.
3. Iber C, Ancoli Israel S, Chesson A, et al, For the American Academy of Sleep Medicine. The AASM manual for the scoring of sleep and associated events. 1st edition. Westchester (IL): American Academy of Sleep medicine; 2007.
4. Malhotra A, Muse VV, Mark EJ. Case records of the Massachusetts General Hospital. Weekly clinicopathological exercises. Case 12-2003. An 82-year-old man with dyspnea and pulmonary abnormalities. N Engl J Med 2003;348:1574–85.
5. Naughton MT, Benard DC, Liu PP, et al. Effects of nasal CPAP on sympathetic activity in patients with heart failure and central sleep apnea. Am J Respir Crit Care Med 1995;152:473–9.
6. Wang H, Parker JD, Newton GE, et al. Influence of obstructive sleep apnea on mortality in patients with heart failure. J Am Coll Cardiol 2007;49: 1625–31.
7. Arzt M, Floras JS, Logan AG, et al. Suppression of central sleep apnea by continuous positive airway pressure and transplant-free survival in heart failure: a post hoc analysis of the Canadian Continuous Positive Airway Pressure for Patients with Central Sleep Apnea and Heart Failure Trial (CANPAP). Circulation 2007;115: 3173–80.
8. Randerath WJ. Therapeutic options for the treatment of Cheyne-Stokes respiration. Swiss Med Wkly 2009;139:135–9.
9. Sasayama S, Izumi T, Seino Y, et al. Effects of nocturnal oxygen therapy on outcome measures in patients with chronic heart failure and Cheyne-Stokes respiration. Circulation 2006;70:1–7.
10. Gold AR, Bleecker ER, Smith PL. A shift from central and mixed sleep apnea to obstructive sleep apnea resulting from low-flow oxygen. Am Rev Respir Dis 1985;132:220–3.

11. White DP, Zwillich CW, Pickett CK, et al. Central sleep apnea. Improvement with acetazolamide therapy. Arch Intern Med 1982;142:1816–9.

12. DeBacker WA, Verbraecken J, Willemen M, et al. Central apnea index decreases after prolonged treatment with acetazolamide. Am J Respir Crit Care Med 1995;151:87–91.

13. Sharp JT, Druz WS, D'Souza V, et al. Effect of metabolic acidosis upon sleep apnea. Chest 1985;87: 619–24.

14. Aurora RN, Chowdhuri S, Ramar K, et al. The treatment of central sleep apnea syndromes in adults: practice parameters with an evidence-based literature review and meta-analyses. Sleep 2012; 35:17–40.

15. Sin DD, Logan AG, Fitzgerald FS, et al. Effects of continuous positive airway pressure on cardiovascular outcomes in heart failure patients with and without Cheyne-Stokes respiration. Circulation 2000;102:61–6.

16. Bradley TD, Logan AG, Kimoff RJ, et al. Continuous positive airway pressure for central sleep apnea and heart failure. N Engl J Med 2005;353:2025–33.

17. Teschler H, Dohring J, Wang YM, et al. Adaptive pressure support servo-ventilation: a novel treatment for Cheyne-Stokes respiration in heart failure. Am J Respir Crit Care Med 2001;164:614–9.

18. Mansfield DR, Gollogly NC, Kaye DM, et al. Controlled trial of continuous positive airway pressure in obstructive sleep apnea and heart failure. Am J Respir Crit Care Med 2004;169:361–6.

19. Javaheri S. Effects of continuous positive airway pressure on sleep apnea and ventricular irritability in patients with heart failure. Circulation 2000;101: 392–7.

20. Naughton MT, Rahman MA, Hara K, et al. Effect of continuous positive airway pressure on intrathoracic and left ventricular transmural pressures in patients with congestive heart failure. Circulation 1995;91:1725–31.

21. Naughton MT, Liu PP, Bernard DC, et al. Treatment of congestive heart failure and Cheyne-Stokes respiration during sleep by continuous positive airway pressure. Am J Respir Crit Care Med 1995;151:92–7.

22. Tkacova R, Hall MJ, Liu PP, et al. Left ventricular volume in patients with heart failure and Cheyne-Stokes respiration during sleep. Am J Respir Crit Care Med 1997;156:1549–55.

23. Kaneko Y, Floras JS, Usui K, et al. Cardiovascular effects of continuous positive airway pressure in patients with heart failure and obstructive sleep apnea. N Engl J Med 2003;348:1233–41.

24. Bradley TD, Holloway RM, McLaughlin PR, et al. Cardiac output response to continuous positive airway pressure in congestive heart failure. Am Rev Respir Dis 1992;145:377–82.

25. Buckle P, Millar T, Kryger M. The effect of short-term nasal CPAP on Cheyne-Stokes respiration in congestive heart failure. Chest 1992;102: 31–5.

26. Davies RJ, Harrington KJ, Ormerod OJ, et al. Nasal continuous positive airway pressure in chronic heart failure with sleep-disordered breathing. Am Rev Respir Dis 1993;147:630–4.

27. Kaye DM, Mansfield D, Aggarwal A, et al. Acute effects of continuous positive airway pressure on cardiac sympathetic tone in congestive heart failure. Circulation 2001;103:2336–8.

28. Malone S, Liu PP, Holloway R, et al. Obstructive sleep apnoea in patients with dilated cardiomyopathy: effects of continuous positive airway pressure. Lancet 1991;338:1480–4.

29. Krachman SL, D'Alonzo GE, Berger TJ, et al. Comparison of oxygen therapy with nasal continuous positive airway pressure on Cheyne-Stokes respiration during sleep in congestive heart failure. Chest 1999;116:1550–7.

30. Arzt M, Wensel R, Montalvan S, et al. Effects of dynamic bilevel positive airway pressure support on central sleep apnea in men with heart failure. Chest 2008;134:61–6.

31. Galetke W, Anduleit N, Kenter M, et al. Evaluation of a new algorithm for patients with Cheyne-Stokes breathing and obstructive sleep apnea. Am J Respir Crit Care Med 2008;177:A480.

32. Javaheri S, Goetting MG, Khayat R, et al. The performance of two automatic servo-ventilation devices in the treatment of central sleep apnea. Sleep 2011;34:1693–8.

33. Randerath WJ. Every cloud has a silver lining—treatment of complicated breathing patterns during sleep. Sleep 2011;34:1625–6.

34. Oldenburg O, Bitter T, Lehmann R, et al. Adaptive servoventilation improves cardiac function and respiratory stability. Clin Res Cardiol 2011;100: 107–15.

35. Johnson KG, Johnson DC. Bilevel positive airway pressure worsens central apneas during sleep. Chest 2005;128:2141–50.

36. Morgenthaler TI, Kagramanov V, Hanak V, et al. Complex sleep apnea syndrome: is it a unique clinical syndrome? Sleep 2006;29:1203–9.

37. Randerath WJ, Galetke W, Stieglitz S, et al. Adaptive servo-ventilation in patients with coexisting obstructive sleep apnoea/hypopnoea and Cheyne-Stokes respiration. Sleep Med 2008;9: 823–30.

38. Kasai T, Usui Y, Yoshioka T, et al. Effect of flow-triggered adaptive servo-ventilation compared with continuous positive airway pressure in patients with chronic heart failure with coexisting obstructive sleep apnea and Cheyne-Stokes respiration. Circ Heart Fail 2010;3:140–8.

39. Randerath WJ, Nothofer G, Priegnitz C, et al. Long-term auto servo-ventilation or constant positive pressure in heart failure and co-existing central with obstructive sleep apnea. Chest 2012;142: 440–7.

40. Arzt M, Schroll S, Series F, et al. Auto-servo ventilation in heart failure with sleep apnea—a randomized controlled trial. Eur Respir J 2013;42:1244–54.

41. Sharma BK, Bakker JP, McSharry DG, et al. Adaptive servoventilation for treatment of sleep-disordered breathing in heart failure: a systematic review and meta-analysis. Chest 2012;142: 1211–21.

42. Hastings PC, Vazir A, Meadows GE, et al. Adaptive servo-ventilation in heart failure patients with sleep apnea: a real world study. Int J Cardiol 2010;139: 17–24.

43. Philippe C, Stoica-Herman M, Drouot X, et al. Compliance with and effectiveness of adaptive ser-voventilation versus continuous positive airway pressure in the treatment of Cheyne-Stokes respiration in heart failure over a six month period. Heart 2006;92:337–42.

44. Yoshihisa A, Shimizu T, Owada T, et al. Adaptive servo ventilation improves cardiac dysfunction and prognosis in chronic heart failure patients with Cheyne-Stokes respiration. Int Heart J 2011; 52:218–23.

45. Koyama T, Watanabe H, Terada S, et al. Adaptive servo-ventilation improves renal function in patients with heart failure. Respir Med 2011;105: 1946–53.

46. Miyata M, Yoshihisa A, Suzuki S, et al. Adaptive servo ventilation improves Cheyne-Stokes respiration, cardiac function, and prognosis in chronic heart failure patients with cardiac resynchronization therapy. J Cardiol 2012;60:222–7.

47. Yamada S, Sakakibara M, Yokota T, et al. Acute hemodynamic effects of adaptive servo-ventilation in patients with heart failure. Circ J 2013;77:1214–20.

48. Pinsky MR, Matuschak GM, Klain M. Determinants of cardiac augmentation by elevations in intrathoracic pressure. J Appl Physiol 1985;58:1189–98.

49. Johnston WE, Vinten-Johansen J, Santamore WP, et al. Mechanism of reduced cardiac output during positive end-expiratory pressure in the dog. Am Rev Respir Dis 1989;140:1257–64.

50. Philip-Joet FF, Paganelli FF, Dutau HL, et al. Hemodynamic effects of bilevel nasal positive airway pressure ventilation in patients with heart failure. Respiration 1999;66:136–43.

51. Haruki N, Takeuchi M, Kaku K, et al. Comparison of acute and chronic impact of adaptive servo-ventilation on left chamber geometry and function in patients with chronic heart failure. Eur J Heart Fail 2011;13:1140–6.

52. Harada D, Joho S, Oda Y, et al. Short term effect of adaptive servo-ventilation on muscle sympathetic nerve activity in patients with heart failure. Auton Neurosci 2011;161:95–102.

53. Pepperell JC, Maskell NA, Jones DR, et al. A randomized controlled trial of adaptive ventilation for Cheyne-Stokes breathing in heart failure. Am J Respir Crit Care Med 2003;168:1109–14.

54. Takama N, Kurabayashi M. Effectiveness of adaptive servo-ventilation for treating heart failure regardless of the severity of sleep-disordered breathing. Circ J 2011;75:1164–9.

55. Koyama T, Watanabe H, Igarashi G, et al. Short-term prognosis of adaptive servo-ventilation therapy in patients with heart failure. Circ J 2011;75: 710–2.

56. Arzt M, Young T, Finn L, et al. Sleepiness and sleep in patients with both systolic heart failure and obstructive sleep apnea. Arch Intern Med 2006; 166:1716–22.

57. Wolkove N, Baltzan M, Kamel H, et al. Long-term compliance with continuous positive airway pressure in patients with obstructive sleep apnea. Can Respir J 2008;15:365–9.

58. Koyama T, Watanabe H, Igarashi G, et al. Effect of short-duration adaptive servo-ventilation therapy on cardiac function in patients with heart failure. Circ J 2012;76:2606–13.

59. Bitter T, Westerheide N, Faber L, et al. Adaptive servoventilation in diastolic heart failure and Cheyne-Stokes respiration. Eur Respir J 2010;36: 385–92.

60. Yoshihisa A, Suzuki S, Miyata M, et al. 'A single night' beneficial effects of adaptive servo-ventilation on cardiac overload, sympathetic nervous activity, and myocardial damage in patients with chronic heart failure and sleep-disordered breathing. Circ J 2012;76:2153–8.

61. Szollosi I, O'Driscoll DM, Dayer MJ, et al. Adaptive servo-ventilation and deadspace: effects on central sleep apnoea. J Sleep Res 2006;15:199–205.

62. Cowie MR, Woehrle H, Wegscheider K, et al. Rationale and design of the SERVE-HF study: treatment of sleep-disordered breathing with predominant central sleep apnoea with adaptive servo-ventilation in patients with chronic heart failure. Eur J Heart Fail 2013;15:937–43.

63. Pusalavidyasagar SS, Olson EJ, Gay PC, et al. Treatment of complex sleep apnea syndrome: a retrospective comparative review. Sleep Med 2006;7:474–9.

64. Badr MS, Toiber F, Skatrud JB, et al. Pharyngeal narrowing/occlusion during central sleep apnea. J Appl Physiol 1995;78:1806–15.

65. Kuzniar TJ, Golbin JM, Morgenthaler TI. Moving beyond empiric continuous positive airway pressure (CPAP) trials for central sleep apnea: a

multi-modality titration study. Sleep Breath 2007; 11:259–66.

66. Morgenthaler TI, Gay PC, Gordon N, et al. Adaptive servoventilation versus noninvasive positive pressure ventilation for central, mixed, and complex sleep apnea syndromes. Sleep 2007;30:468–75.

67. Allam JS, Olson EJ, Gay PC, et al. Efficacy of adaptive servoventilation in treatment of complex and central sleep apnea syndromes. Chest 2007;132: 1839–46.

68. Carnevale C, Georges M, Rabec C, et al. Effectiveness of adaptive servo ventilation in the treatment of hypocapnic central sleep apnea of various etiologies. Sleep Med 2011;12:952–8.

69. Randerath WJ, George S. Opioid-induced sleep apnea: is it a real problem? J Clin Sleep Med 2012;8:577–8.

70. Kelly LE, Rieder M, van den Anker J, et al. More codeine fatalities after tonsillectomy in North American children. Pediatrics 2012;129:e1343–7.

71. Walker JM, Farney RJ, Rhondeau SM, et al. Chronic opioid use is a risk factor for the development of central sleep apnea and ataxic breathing. J Clin Sleep Med 2007;3:455–61.

72. Pattinson KT. Opioids and the control of respiration. Br J Anaesth 2008;100:747–58.

73. Farney RJ, Walker JM, Boyle KM, et al. Adaptive servoventilation (ASV) in patients with sleep disordered breathing associated with chronic opioid medications for non-malignant pain. J Clin Sleep Med 2008;4:311–9.

74. Javaheri S, Malik A, Smith J, et al. Adaptive pressure support servoventilation: a novel treatment for sleep apnea associated with use of opioids. J Clin Sleep Med 2008;4:305–10.

75. Ramar K, Ramar P, Morgenthaler TI. Adaptive servoventilation in patients with central or complex sleep apnea related to chronic opioid use and congestive heart failure. J Clin Sleep Med 2012;8: 569–76.

Alternative Approaches to Treatment of Central Sleep Apnea

Robert Joseph Thomas, MD, MMSc

KEYWORDS

- Carbon dioxide • Oxygen rebreathing • Acetazolamide • Provent • Winx • Multimodal complex
- Central apnea • Periodic breathing

KEY POINTS

- The phenotype that reflects heightened respiratory chemoreflex activation is non–rapid eye movement (NREM)-dominant sleep apnea. Conventional scoring may categorize many of these patients as obstructive.
- Targeting respiratory chemoreflex sensitivity or effects, and sleep fragmentation, can provide useful alternative or adjunctive therapy for central sleep apnea syndromes.
- CO_2 is the dominant driver of sleep respiration, and manipulation of CO_2 has the greatest potential for clinical effects. The primary challenges are simultaneously technical and biological: how to keep the CO_2 levels just above the NREM sleep CO_2 threshold. As these levels are not hypercapnic, sympathoexcitation would not occur.
- Treatments for obstructive components of sleep apnea that may be less prone to destabilize respiratory control include Provent, oral appliances, and Winx. However, residual disease is common and requires adjunctive therapies.
- Reducing the impact of arousals and inducing a stable form of NREM sleep may be achieved by sedatives, including the classic benzodiazepines and the nonbenzodiazepines such as zolpidem.
- Multimodality approaches to the treatment of sleep apnea are especially important for central sleep apnea syndromes.

INTRODUCTION

The treatment of central sleep apnea syndromes, especially the hypocapnic type characterized by a hyperactive respiratory chemoreflex, is challenging. The adaptive servoventilators target respiratory rhythm besides providing upper airway support, and are described in other articles in this issue. In this article alternative approaches to management are described, which in some instances may be used as adjuncts to positive airway pressure (PAP). As the hypocapnic central sleep apnea syndromes are characterized by specific pathologic rhythms of respiration, accurate polysomnographic recognition of driving chemoreflex influences is critical in dosing primary and adjunctive/alternative therapies. Phenotyping of

Disclosures: Dr Thomas is: (1) coinventor of the ECG-spectrogram technique to phenotype sleep and sleep apnea. This technology is licensed by the Beth Israel Deaconess Medical Center to MyCardio, LLC; (2) coinventor of the Positive Airway Pressure Gas Modulator, a device that treats central/complex apnea with low concentration CO_2 added to positive pressure therapy. He consults for DeVilbiss in the development of a new-generation auto-CPAP.
Division of Pulmonary, Critical Care & Sleep, Department of Medicine, Beth Israel Deaconess Medical Center, Harvard Medical School, 330 Brookline Avenue, Boston, MA 02215, USA
E-mail address: rthomas1@bidmc.harvard.edu

Sleep Med Clin 9 (2014) 87–104
http://dx.doi.org/10.1016/j.jsmc.2013.10.008
1556-407X/14/$ – see front matter © 2014 Elsevier Inc. All rights reserved.

the contributory components of sleep apnea is central to phenotype-driven therapy. The phenotypes that have current treatment options are upper airway collapsibility, chemoreflex activation level, and sleep fragmentation propensity.

POLYSOMNOGRAPHIC RECOGNITION OF A HEIGHTENED RESPIRATORY CHEMOREFLEX

Scoring of respiratory events in sleep apnea patients have traditionally been biased toward an obstructive phenotype, although the recent update of the 2007 American Academy of Sleep Medicine (AASM) guidelines has criteria for scoring central hypopneas and short sequences of periodic breathing/Cheyne-Stokes respiration.[1] The guidelines state that central hypopneas should not be scored in the presence of flow limitation, but obstruction is a common feature of central events,[2] even at simulated altitude,[3] the latter being a relatively pure model of chemoreflex-driven sleep apnea. Direct visualization of the upper airway shows collapse at the nadir of the cycle to be common even in polysomnographic central disease.[4] Expiratory pharyngeal narrowing occurs during central hypocapnic hypopnea,[5] directly supporting the concept that the presence of flow limitation alone cannot be used to distinguish obstructive and central hypopneas.[3] Complex sleep apnea as currently defined requires a central apnea-hypopnea index (AHI; number of apneas and hypopneas per hour of sleep) of 5 or more, with centrally mediated respiratory events constituting 50% or more of all respiratory events during continuous positive airway pressure (CPAP) titration, in those who do not fulfill criteria for primary central sleep apnea or periodic breathing on the diagnostic polysomnogram. However, publications of complex apnea did not score central hypopneas or periodic breathing. Descriptions of low (<5%) persistence of complex apnea may be inaccurate and reflect reliance solely on scoring classic central apneas.[6,7] The guideline for recognition of Cheyne-Stokes respiration also require a cycle duration of at least 40 seconds, but the author has shown that even shorter cycle times in the range of 20 to 25 seconds is typical of non–rapid eye movement (NREM)-dominant sleep apnea,[8] reminiscent of high-altitude periodic breathing. The most characteristic feature of chemoreflex-driven events is not the morphology of individual events but NREM dominance and timing/morphology of sequential events (nearly identical) in a consecutive series of events.[9]

A related dimension is the criteria used for estimating success of therapies. For example, if 4% oxygen desaturation is used to score hypopneas (used in most treatment reports, and which continues to be the recommendation of the AASM), significant degrees of baseline and residual disease can be missed. Moreover, adaptive servoventilators distort the conventional polysomnogram signals and, unless the pressure output of the devices are used to score events, inappropriate success may be declared. When periodic breathing is not adequately controlled, the primary marker on the polysomnogram is pressure cycling associated with arousals. Scoring respiratory events during adaptive servoventilation needs to use the pressure output signal from the ventilator, which is roughly equal and opposite to the patient's abnormality. When pressure cycling persists, sleep fragmentation is usually severe even if respiration is improved by conventional criteria.

ADVANCED PHENOTYPING OF CHEMOREFLEX INFLUENCES ON SLEEP RESPIRATION

The NREM sleep CO_2 reserve can be exposed inadvertently during bilevel positive pressure titration in the sleep laboratory, when central apneas or periodic breathing may emerge even if continuous positive pressure is well tolerated and efficacious. An experimentally precise version of this approach uses bilevel ventilation with measurement of end-tidal CO_2 ($ETCO_2$), the difference between stable breathing and the level just before bilevel-induced periodic breathing or central apneas. The CO_2 reserve is smaller (2–3 mm Hg) in those with heart failure and predominantly central sleep apnea.[10] Proportional assist ventilation may also be used to estimate the ease of induction of central apnea and periodic breathing, and thus quantify the contribution of enhanced respiratory chemoreflexes to sleep apnea severity.[11–15] This technique requires considerable expertise and is not readily applicable to a clinical laboratory environment.

Time series analysis of the electrocardiogram (ECG) (using heart-rate variability and heart rate/respiratory coupling) can provide a map of sleep-state oscillations, with the spectral dispersion providing phenotyping information regarding chemoreflex influences.[9] The technique, the ECG-spectrogram, maps coupled oscillations of heart-rate variability and respiratory R-wave ECG amplitude modulation. The ECG-derived sleep spectrogram can detect low-frequency coupled oscillations with 2 primary patterns: broad band and narrow band. Elevated narrow-band coupling, which detects sequences of central apneas and periodic breathing, is noted in patients with complex sleep apnea. Those with the ECG-spectrogram biomarker of strong chemoreflex modulation of sleep respiration also have more severe sleep apnea and greater degrees of sleep fragmentation.[16] A wearable device, the M1, approval by the Food and Drug Administration (www.sleepimage.com) is currently available for clinical and research use.

Determination of multiple phenotypic traits can be accomplished by assessing the dynamic flow and pressure responses to positive pressure dial down.[17] In a follow-up study,[18] 75 men and women aged 20 to 65 years with and without obstructive sleep apnea (OSA) were studied on 3 separate nights. Anatomic collapsibility (Pcrit) and nonanatomic factors (genioglossus muscle responsiveness, arousal threshold, and respiratory control stability/loop gain) were determined. The key findings, varied substantially between participants. In brief, 36% of OSA patients had minimal genioglossus muscle responsiveness during sleep, 37% had a low arousal threshold, 36% had high loop gain, and 28% had multiple nonanatomic features. Nineteen percent had a relatively noncollapsible upper airway similar to controls, and in these patients loop gain was almost twice as high as that in patients with a collapsible airway, despite comparable AHI.

Experimental elegance does not readily translate to clinical utility. However, review of the data tables of virtually all publications on central and complex sleep apnea, regardless of exact criteria and comorbid diseases such as congestive heart failure, and when available in description of sleep apnea phenotyping approaches, show one common theme: NREM sleep dominance of sleep apnea. **Table 1** describes the features of an activated respiratory chemoreflex on polysomnographic and polygraphic (eg, home sleep studies) assessments. These features are valid on diagnostic assessments and during therapeutic interventions. **Figs. 1** and **2** show an overall schema of integration of various therapeutic modalities with and without PAP, respectively.

NON–POSITIVE AIRWAY PRESSURE TREATMENTS FOR CENTRAL SLEEP APNEA SYNDROMES
Minimization of Hypocapnia

The use of supplemental CO_2 for hypocapnic central sleep apnea syndromes is old news. That CO_2 can stabilize respiration has been known for decades, but high concentrations fragment sleep by inducing arousals secondary to respiratory stimulation and sympathoexcitation.[19,20] The key challenge has been delivery of CO_2 in a clinically adequate, tolerated, and precise manner. Prevention of hypocapnia is a critical stabilizing

factor in sleep respiratory control. Minimization of hypocapnia is also physiologically a more appropriate phrase than induction of hypercapnia, as the latter is utterly unnecessary. The key is holding the CO_2 steady and just above the NREM sleep CO_2 threshold, thus protecting the CO_2 reserve.

A recent study by Xie and colleagues[21] is one of the best demonstrations of the power of CO_2 modulation in treating sleep apnea syndromes. Twenty-six patients with OSA (AHI 42 $\pm$ 5 events/h with 92% of apnea being obstructive) were treated with O_2 supplementation, an isocapnic rebreathing system in which CO_2 was added only during hyperpnea to prevent transient hypocapnia, using a continuous rebreathing system. Each patient's controller gain below eupnea was measured, as was CO_2 reserve, plant gain, and passive upper airway closing pressure. With isocapnic rebreathing, 14 of 26 patients reduced their AHI to 31% $\pm$ 6% of control ($P<.01$) (responders); 12 of 26 did not show significant change (nonresponders). Compared with nonresponders, the responders had a greater controller gain, a smaller CO_2 reserve, but no differences in Pcrit. Hypercapnic rebreathing (+4.2 $\pm$ 1 mm Hg ETCO$_2$ pressure [PETCO$_2$]) reduced AHI to 15% $\pm$ 4% of control ($P<.001$) in 17 of 21 subjects with a wide range of CO_2 reserve. Hyperoxia (arterial oxygen saturation $\sim$95%–98%) reduced AHI to 36% $\pm$ 11% of control in 7 of 19 OSA patients tested.

Thus, there is strong evidence from multiple studies over the years that manipulation of arterial CO_2 levels might provide an alternative treatment strategy. Addition of a closed volume (space) to exhalation increases rebreathing of the exhaled air, and results in a quick increase in CO_2 levels and an increased tidal volume and respiratory rate. This process is similar to breathing into a plastic bag when trying to treat anxiety-induced hyperventilation. Increased amounts (>300 mL) manifestly feel uncomfortable from both CO_2 retention and volume effects. The concept has been used for several years in mechanical ventilation to reduce hypocapnia, and more recently has been successfully used to treat central sleep apnea and Cheyne-Stokes respiration in heart failure. None of these uses combine it with PAP.

The author's group has shown that keeping CO_2 above the apnea threshold with the use of enhanced expiratory rebreathing space (EERS) is an effective adjunct to PAP therapy.[22] EERS is the dead-space concept applied to pressure ventilation. PAP therapy usually induces mild relative (to pretreatment) hypocapnia. Central apneas and periodic breathing can be generated when the

Table 1
Recognition of strong chemoreflex modulation of sleep-breathing

Polysomnographic Characteristic	Relatively Pure Obstructive Sleep Apnea	Chemoreflex-Modulated Sleep Apnea
Obstructive apneas	Dominant	Less common
Central apneas	Rare	Dominant form of apneas
Progressive flow limitation	Typical; long variable-length segments of limited breaths are typical	Commonly seen with mixed apneas except for in the purest form (eg, in classic Cheyne-Stokes respiration)
Periodic breathing/Cheyne-Stokes pattern	Rare; may be seen at sleep onset or around sleep-wake transitions	Typical (often short cycle, $\leq$30 s, in the absence of congestive heart failure)
Relative severity in NREM vs REM sleep	Greater severity in REM sleep	Minimal severity in REM sleep; this may be best evident during CPAP titrations
Positive pressure therapy	Generally good response with improvement in flow limitation and AHI	Response variable; may worsen with positive pressure therapy
Central apneas before elimination of flow limitation during titration	Rare	Typical
Respiratory event cycle durations	Variable	Short cycle (25–35 s) is highly suggestive, but long cycle forms also occur
Respiratory event symmetry in NREM sleep including a mirror-imaging pattern	Minimal symmetry	Very symmetric, and mirror imaging is typical (one half of an event is the mirror image of the other)
Effort signal morphology	Well maintained during obstructed breath	Complete or partial loss between recovery breath clusters
Flow-effort relationships	Discordant: flow is reduced disproportionately to reduction in effort signals	Concordant: flow and effort follow each other in amplitude
Arousal timing	Early part of event termination, often first recovery breath related	Crests event, often in the center of a sequence of recovery breaths that progressively increase in amplitude and decrease
Oxygen desaturation profile	Irregular, progressive drops, sharp contour (V shape)	Smooth, symmetric, progressive drops rare. Rarely <80% (band pattern)
CO_2	If CO_2 is affected, generally eupneic or hypercapnic	Usually hypocapnic
Nonadaptive bilevel PAP-induced instability	Less common, usually with excessive pressure support or severe mask leak only	Typical

Abbreviations: AHI, apnea-hypopnea index; CPAP, continuous positive airway pressure; NREM, non–rapid eye movement; PAP, positive airway pressure; REM, rapid eye movement.

level of arterial pressure of CO_2 falls below that required to stimulate respiration. This level is referred to as the apnea threshold. Hypocapnia at or near the apnea or CO_2 control threshold destabilizes sleep-breathing control, resulting in periodic breathing patterns of various severities and morphologic characteristics. Preventing hypocapnia is a powerful stabilizing influence on

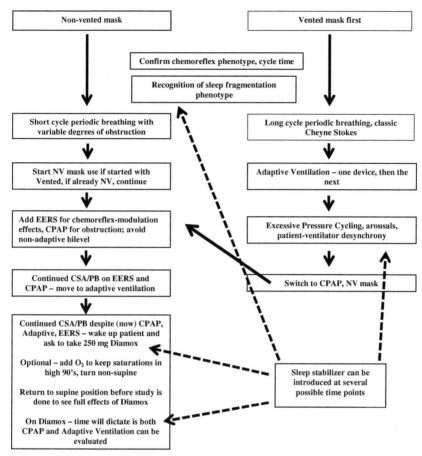

Fig. 1. How to use alternative and adjunctive therapies for central sleep apnea: positive airway pressure (PAP)-based approaches. CPAP, continuous positive airway pressure; CSA, central sleep apnea; EERS, enhanced expiratory rebreathing space; NV, nonvented; PB, periodic breathing.

sleep-breathing control, regardless of the presence of hypoxia. Atmospheric CO_2 levels are near zero, therefore the CO_2 levels in the blood are the result of the balance between metabolism in the patient and blow-off during breathing.

The clinical effect of using EERS is consistently positive (**Fig. 3**), and this approach is now routinely available in the author's sleep laboratory for use with CPAP or adaptive servoventilation, as requested by the physician. In the original report the author's group[22] described improved clinical tolerance, compliance, and sustained clinical improvement monitored over a period of several months by adding EERS, achieved in a subgroup of patients who had stopped using CPAP and were salvaged with the use of EERS. Subtidal volume dead space is adequate when the upper airway is also supported, and is well tolerated physiologically. Control of respiratory abnormality is achieved with minimal increase in CO_2 (2–3 mm Hg) which, judging by the beneficial

effects seen within 20 to 30 seconds, is speculated to be due to the effect on carotid chemoreceptors.

There is strictly no true dead space when this concept is used with pressure ventilation. Mixing, turbulence, and leaks ensure variable degrees of effective rebreathing (hence the suggested term enhanced expiratory rebreathing space). There is, however, a reduction in ventilatory blow-off, with remarkable clinical effectiveness. There is no minimal increase in inspiratory CO_2 because of the positive pressure–induced washout. One important practical effect of using PAP with EERS is that the respiratory rate seems unchanged, and the subject does not notice any significant discomfort. This fact is not surprising, given the known effects of positive pressure support on relieving shortness of breath in mechanically ventilated patients. Such symptom minimization is obviously important when considering the use of EERS in patients who are already short of breath, such as in those with heart failure.

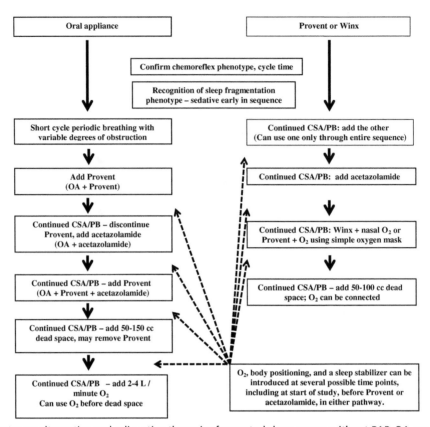

Fig. 2. How to use alternative and adjunctive therapies for central sleep apnea without PAP. OA, oral appliance.

The physiologic target for titrations with EERS is to maintain ETCO$_2$ within the low normal range for sleep. Normal sleep results in an increase of 2 to 8 mm Hg in ETCO$_2$. With this technique the target is to keep the ETCO$_2$ in the high 30s to low 40s, the lower end of normal. Those with central and mixed sleep-disordered breathing show a prominent tendency to hypocapnia during sleep. The primary monitoring is that of ETCO$_2$ with a mainstream CO$_2$ sensor at the mask. Transcutaneous CO$_2$ may usefully complement end-tidal measures, but is not critical for the treatment of hypocapnic central/complex sleep apnea. Transcutaneous measurements can have a role in the management of hypercapnic central apnea. A biocalibration of ETCO$_2$ may be done before the sleep study (1–2 minutes rested steady breathing, average final 10 breaths), with a nonvented (NV) mask and 50, 100, and 150 mL added dead space. This biocalibration may be used to determine the starting EERS volume or to flag those with too high an ETCO$_2$ to use an NV mask approach. The CO$_2$ targets are to keep the ETCO$_2$ below 50 mm Hg during sleep and not greater than 5 mm Hg increase from wake. If transcutaneous CO$_2$ is monitored it should be kept at less than

50 mm Hg, or increases limited to 5 mm Hg from baseline. The latter approach is approximate, because sleep baseline ETCO$_2$ without an NV mask on the patient will probably not be known, and it is unclear how much time is required for equilibration after sleep onset.

The mask-fitting clinic at the Beth Israel Deaconess Medical Center has modified a large number of masks. Specific masks, methods to convert to NV, and appropriate connectors are available on request (contact the author at rthomas1@bidmc.harvard.edu) and are tabulated with mask-specific PowerPoint files. The NV configuration, including the safety valve, adds 60 to 100 mL of dead space (including the intramask space), and this NV alone usually means about 60 to 100 mL of dead space/EERS in comparison with a vented mask. In practical terms this means that adding further EERS is often no longer necessary.

There are 2 approaches to titration of EERS, forward and backward. In the forward approach, incremental options are considered with PAP first with a vented mask, then conversion to an NV mask, then addition of rebreathing space (eg, 50 mL O$_2$, then 100 mL O$_2$, and so forth). In the backward approach, maximal stabilization is

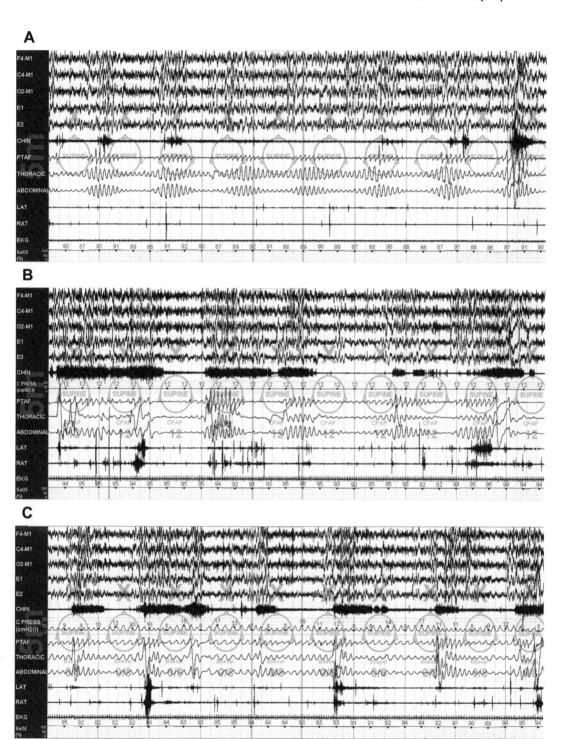

Fig. 3. (*A*) Classic periodic breathing/Cheyne-Stokes respiration (CSR). A 72-year-old with congestive heart failure. Note the typical waxing-waning respiratory pattern. All subsets are from the same patient. (*B*) CSR with CPAP failure. Note continuing CSR. (*C*) CSR with adaptive servoventilation failure. Note excessive cycling of pressure (the CPRESS channel) and the associated arousals. (*D*) CSR with 50 mL enhanced expiratory rebreathing space (EERS). Note stabilization of respiratory rhythm but residual flow limitation and mild residual periodic breathing. (*E*) CSR with 100 mL EERS. Note normalization of sleep and respiration. The end-tidal CO_2 (ETCO$_2$) signal plateau is slightly blunted and thus the CO_2 measured is falsely low. However, the resting wake ETCO$_2$ of this patient was 30 mm Hg, a level that can be readily seen in patients with congestive heart failure.

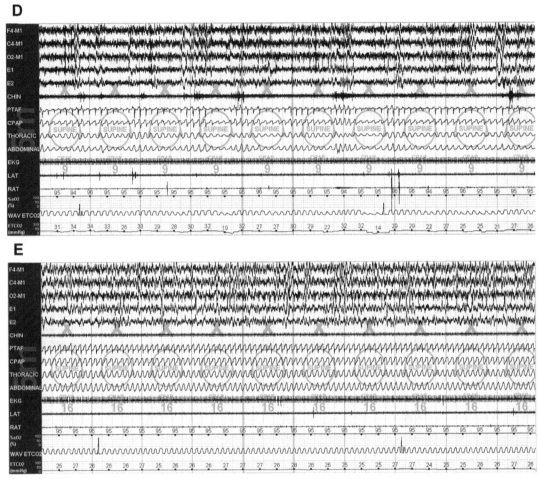

Fig. 3. (*continued*)

provided at the outset, starting at 50 mL dead space (which seems to be adequate for most) and 2 L/min O_2. After obtaining control in rapid eye movement (REM)/stable and unstable NREM sleep, the O_2 and CO_2 modulations can be progressively withdrawn to assess the minimum requirement. Typically with successful dead space, O_2 is not critical but can be a useful backup, because consistently good seals are difficult to maintain at home. Obtaining a plateau on the ETCO$_2$ signal ensures effectiveness (ie, that the seal is adequate) and accuracy of the reading. An alternative approach is to simply start with an NV mask and no added EERS, and titrate as required.

CO$_2$ manipulation can also be done by bleeding CO_2 into the circuit using a more precisely controlled flow-independent method. Successful treatment of mixed obstructive and central sleep apnea using a proprietary device, the PAP gas modulator (PAPGAM), has been reported, which

delivers precisely controlled concentrations of CO_2. In a small case series, 6 patients with average AHI of 43/h on CPAP improved with reduction of AHI to 4.5/h with addition of 0.5% to 1% using PAPGAM.[23] However, this requires experienced technologists and the development of a clinically safe device. Whether dynamic CO_2 manipulation (delivery restricted to a specific phase of the respiratory cycle) will improve on the stabilizing effects of CO_2 is unclear, but if a medical-grade CO_2 source (cylinder) is needed, improved efficiency and duration of a single refill may be achieved.[24]

Oxygen

Nasal O_2 has a long history of use in the treatment of central sleep apnea and periodic breathing.[25,26] Effectiveness is partial, and residual sleep apnea and sleep fragmentation are typical. Adding oxygen to CPAP may result in better control of central/complex apnea, with a reduction in responsiveness of peripheral chemoreceptors and the loop gain.[27] The limitations include the long-term cost and difficulty with reimbursement in nonhypoxic patients. A recent study in a Veterans' population showed that O_2 has beneficial effects, although the polysomnographic changes were delayed by as much as an hour or more.[28] One change to be aware of concerns the length of respiratory event cycle, which can lengthen with the use of O_2. Such a change may reduce the respiratory event index but does not imply a true stabilization of respiration. Use of O_2 also negates the use of a desaturation link to score hypopneas. It should be noted that hypoxia levels used to initiate O_2 therapy are not the threshold for evaluating supplemental O_2; moving saturations from the mid-90s to the high 90s can be beneficial. Use of O_2 is off-label for central apnea syndromes. Supplemental O_2 can thus be a useful component of a multimodal, multistep approach to the management of central sleep apnea syndromes. **Fig. 4** is an example of the use of supplemental O_2 during positive pressure therapy, along with EERS. The treatment response also provides information about the phenotype.

Sleep Stabilization

Most patients, including older individuals or those on benzodiazepines/sedative drugs, exhibit periods of sleep that are not scored as N3 by conventional criteria (or any modification thereof), but clearly have ample low-amplitude delta frequency waves. Respiration is usually fairly stable during this period (functionally considered as slow-wave sleep) and, if recognized, the same precautions as used during conventionally scored slow-wave sleep apply. Those who study the cyclic alternating pattern (CAP) will recognize this type of stable NREM sleep as predominantly non-CAP.[29] In fact, for the purpose of titration, dividing sleep into stable and unstable NREM sleep (or non-CAP/CAP) and REM works well, more so than N1 to N3 and REM sleep. It may be easier to recognize stable and unstable NREM sleep from non-electroencephalographic (EEG) signals, such as respiration, heart-rate variability, and respiratory amplitude modulation of the ECG.[30] The stability of this non-CAP or slow-wave–like (frequency but not amplitude) sleep can cause a false sense of security (of treatment efficacy); it is also important not to change pressures if this state is recognized (unless obstructions and flow limitation are overt). Flow can look absolutely normal in this state, but rather abruptly (often within a minute) a switch to being abnormal

may occur. Such switches of stable/unstable state are spontaneous, and disease or treatment needs to deal with this dynamic.

The sleep-fragmentation phenotype can be suggested by several polysomnographic features. There may be prolonged (>5–10 minutes) sleep-wake transitional instability. The same pattern can be seen if the laboratory bedtime is before the internal biological night (a phase-delayed person trying to sleep hours before natural bedtime). The sleep efficiency may be low (less than 70%) and stage N1 remaining increased (>15%) during the positive pressure titration study. There may be prolonged postarousal instability (1–2 minutes of periodic breathing after individual arousals). Slow waves may evolve poorly across the night with a low density of the waves of slow oscillation (<1 Hz). This process may be more readily visualized than quantitatively estimated in the sleep laboratory, as conventional slow-wave sleep is only a fraction of stable NREM sleep. However, relative paucity of non-CAP EEG morphology during titration (<30%) is a marker the author has found useful. If the fragmentation phenotype is recognized, the options are: (1) reduce pressure (watch for evidence of increased obstruction) or change mode; (2) allow the patient to take a break, until subjective sleepiness is noted, to allow better expression of homeostatic sleep drive; (3) trigger the physician-directed drug option if ordered.

The core concept then is to use sedatives that can induce stable NREM sleep. Whereas the conventional approach avoids sedatives in OSA, these drugs can be used safely for NREM-dominant apnea, in which arousals further destabilize sleep and worsen the severity of sleep apnea. In fact, eszopiclone can improve sleep apnea in those with a low arousal threshold.[31] Arousals from sleep and frequent sleep-stage transitions can both induce and increase the severity of central and complex sleep apnea. The proposed mechanisms are arousal-induced hypocapnia, reduction of upper airway resistance on arousal, and increased neural output to respiratory centers when awake. Triazolam, temazepam, zolpidem, and clonazepam have all been shown to reduce central apnea abnormality.[32–35] The author selectively uses hypnotics, with good clinical results in patients with the sleep-fragmentation phenotype. Short-acting sedatives can be part of a laboratory pharmacology protocol (see **Figs. 1** and **2**), or the patient can take the drug at bedtime.

Reduction of Opioid Dose

Opioid use is a risk factor for the development of ataxic breathing and central sleep apneas.[36–38]

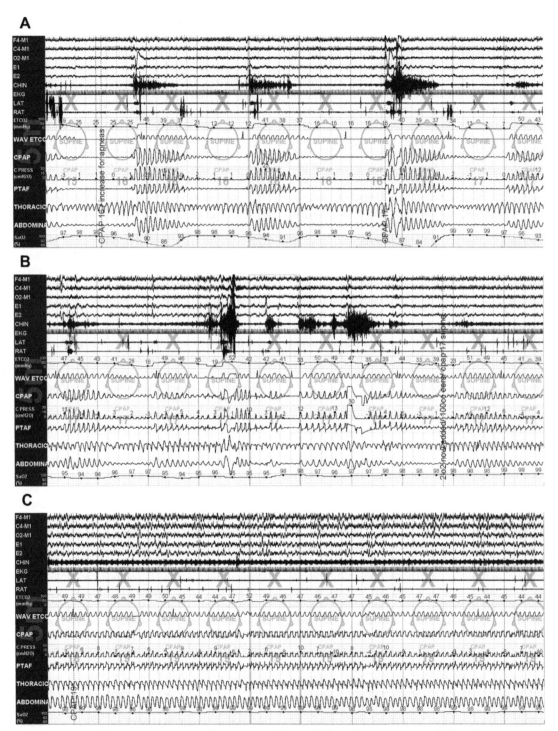

Fig. 4. (*A*) CPAP refractory mixed apnea: obstruction and periodic breathing. Note periodic breathing pattern of respiratory effort, unresponsiveness to CPAP of 16 to 17 cm H_2O, while on a nonvented mask alone without EERS. (*B*) CPAP refractory mixed apnea: CO_2 effects. The same patient as in *A*, but now with 100 mL EERS. Note improved respiratory stabilization, but periodic breathing and obstructive features (flow limitation) coexist and contribute to ongoing sleep fragmentation. (*C*) CPAP refractory mixed apnea: adjunctive O_2 effects. The same patient as in *A*, now with 4 L/min of supplemental oxygen. Note complete stabilization of respiratory rhythm but residual obstruction, which ultimately required 22 cm H_2O to eliminate.

Decreasing the dose of opiates may help reduce central apneas.[39] In most patients stopping opiates entirely is not possible. The pathophysiology involves modulation of hypoxic and hypercapnic ventilatory responses,[40] but opiate receptors are seen throughout the respiratory control pathways. Opiate-induced ataxic breathing is fairly sensitive to CO_2 levels, with ready induction of central apnea and worsening of dysrhythmic breathing with continuous or nonadaptive bilevel positive pressure ventilation. Although these patients tend to show mild hypercapnia, with $ETCO_2$ in the high 40s to low 50s, using an NV mask and EERS as needed to hold CO_2 in the mid-40s can be useful. The author has found the use of acetazolamide to be of consistent benefit. Adaptive servoventilation is a double-edged sword in these patients, being able to both enable stable breathing and markedly destabilize breathing.

Carbonic Anhydrase Inhibition

Acetazolamide, a diuretic and carbonic anhydrase inhibitor, diminishes the ventilatory response of the peripheral chemoreceptors to hypoxia, decreases loop gain, and reduces the ventilatory response to arousals.[41–44] In animal models, it has been shown to lower the $PETCO_2$ apnea threshold and widen the difference between the eupneic and $PETCO_2$ thresholds.[45] Acetazolamide has been used in treating central apneas and Cheyne-Stokes breathing in patients with and without congestive heart failure.[46] Although the results may be statistically significant, the degree of residual sleep apnea is unacceptable as sole long-term therapy. The drug can convert those with mixed obstructive and central sleep apnea to mostly obstructive (the reverse of CPAP-induced central sleep apnea). The drug is now part of the author's algorithm for the management of central sleep

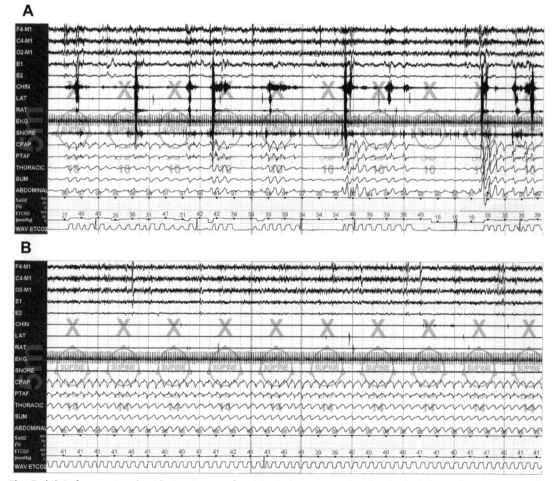

Fig. 5. (A) Before acetazolamide treatment of resistant sleep apnea. At the start of this polysomnogram, the patient was failing CPAP, 150 mL EERS, and supplemental O_2. (B) Post-acetazolamide effects, 1 hour later. The patient received a single dose of 250 mg acetazolamide about 2 hours before this snapshot. Note the complete resolution of central sleep apnea, which was maintained for the rest of the night. 50 mL of EERS was continued.

apnea and periodic breathing. Those with short-cycle (≤30 seconds) periodic breathing not responding to EERS are the best candidates, as in this subset the time constant of the adaptive servo-ventilators seems too long to optimally entrain and stabilize respiration. Carbonic anhydrase inhibition with acetazolamide or topiramate can be part of a laboratory pharmacology protocol, and can be used with an NV mask/EERS (**Fig. 5**). Acetazolamide has been successfully used as CPAP adjuncts at high altitude.[47,48] Zonisamide[49] and topiramate[50] have carbonic anhydrase inhibitory

effects, and could in theory be used in the place of acetazolamide. It is not known whether the neuronal effects would have an impact on integration of respiratory control.

Clonidine

One report describes a potential role for clonidine as adjunctive therapy for hypocapnic central sleep apnea syndromes.[51] In a study of 10 healthy subjects (4 females) (age 22.3 ± 3.0 years; body mass index 25.5 ± 3.4 kg/m²), subjects were

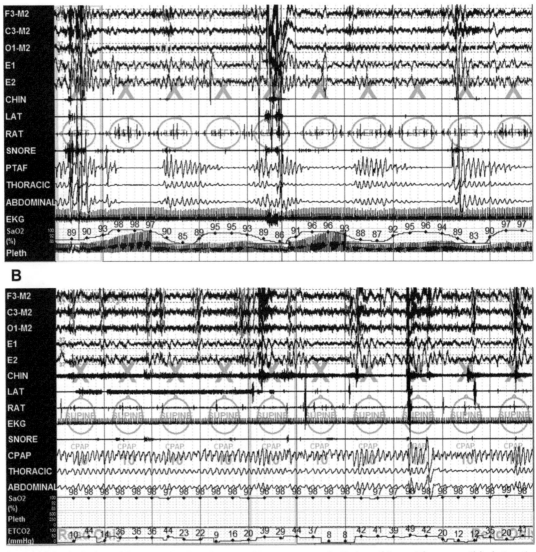

Fig. 6. (A) Periodic breathing, pre-CPAP or Provent. Note severe periodic breathing with some mild obstructive features. (B) Periodic breathing on CPAP in the same patient as in A. Although there is significant improvement in respiration, treatment was not tolerated for home use and there is ongoing clear evidence of sleep fragmentation/arousals. (C) Periodic breathing resolved on Provent in the same patient as in A and B. Note the complete resolution of sleep apnea and absence of arousals.

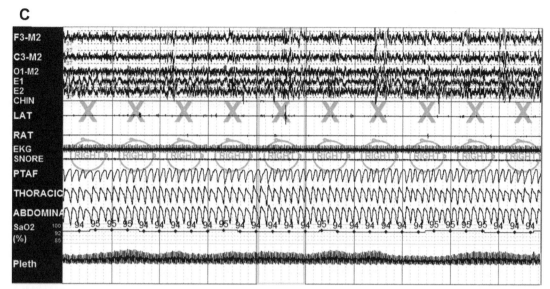

Fig. 6. (*continued*)

randomized to receive placebo or 0.1 mg/45 kg of clonidine on 2 separate nights. Ventilation and upper airway resistance were monitored during wakefulness and sleep. Two separate experiments were performed. In one (8 subjects), CO_2 reserve, hypocapnic apneic threshold, and hypocapnic ventilatory responses were determined using noninvasive hyperventilation to induce hypocapnia. In a second protocol, peripheral hypocapnic ventilatory response was determined by noninvasive ventilation using short (3 breaths) hyperventilation. Clonidine decreased the systolic blood pressure by 12 ± 10 mm Hg but did not affect baseline ventilation or upper airway resistance during wakefulness or sleep. Clonidine was associated with a decreased hypocapnic apneic threshold relative to placebo (37.3 ± 3.3 vs 39.7 ± 3.4 mm Hg), increased CO_2 reserve (-3.8 ± 1.3 vs -2.8 ± 1.2 mm Hg), and decreased hypocapnic ventilatory responses (1.6 ± 0.6 vs 2.5 ± 1.3 L/min/mm Hg). Administration of clonidine did not decrease peripheral ventilatory responses. The hypotensive effect will likely reduce enthusiasm for clinical use, but the concept has merit.

Nasal Expiratory Positive Pressure

Nasal expiratory PAP (Provent; Ventus Medical, San José, CA), another device with a simple design marketed for use in patients with mild OSA, may also be useful in treating central and complex apnea. This device helps generate auto positive end-expiratory pressure and increased tracheal tug via increased lung volumes, which may relieve OSA, but efficacy is variable and unpredictable[52]; in the author's center, about 25% of subjects show acceptable benefits when evaluated during polysomnography, including those with central sleep apnea and periodic breathing (**Fig. 6**). This effect of Provent can be enhanced by acetazolamide, similarly to the use of the drug with CPAP.[48] The author speculates that Provent, while providing increased nasal expiratory resistance also gently increases the $ETCO_2$, which may stabilize the chemoreflex-driven breathing instability.[52]

Oral Appliances

In patients who choose oral appliances as first-line treatment, it is important to be aware that central apneas can also emerge in these settings.[53] The author has used these devices in PAP-intolerant complex apnea patients with reasonable success. Residual sleep apnea is typical, and requires adjunctive therapy. Oral appliances are less likely, it seems, to induce hypocapnia, but treatment of obstruction is less precise. Cocktails that are currently being used include oral appliance + acetazolamide, or a benzodiazepine, or supplemental oxygen. One specific use of an oral appliance is with positive pressure, to reduce pressure requirements.[54,55]

Weight Reduction

Major weight reduction, for example through gastric bypass procedures, can have profound effects on sleep apnea, although true cures are rare. In the author's experience, a small subset of postbypass patients experience conversion of

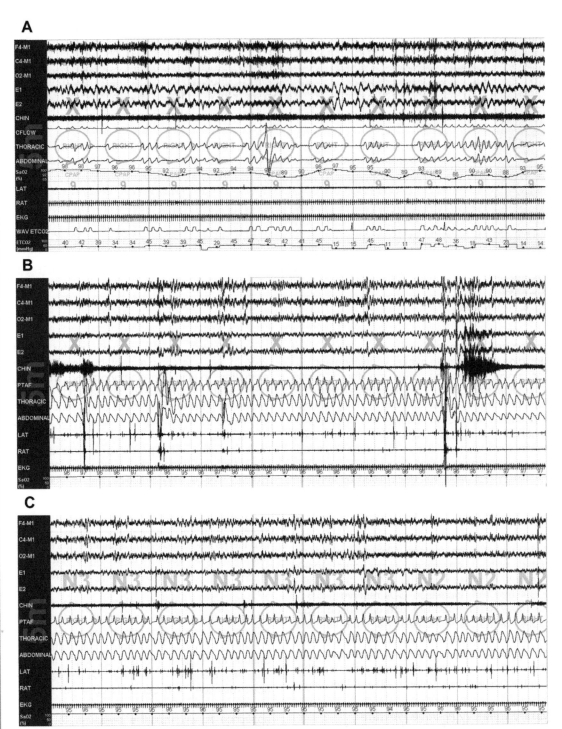

Fig. 7. (*A*) CPAP failure, central sleep apnea. The patient was pretreated with acetazolamide and clonazepam, as there were multiple past failures of positive pressure titration caused by both periodic breathing and severe sleep fragmentation, which was considered disproportionate to the severity of sleep apnea. (*B*) CPAP failure, improved on Winx, in the same patient as in *A*. Note a marked improvement of sleep apnea on Winx, with the residual abnormality seemingly flow limitation and arousals. The relative efficacy of Winx versus CPAP may reflect the tendency of CPAP to worsen hypocapnia. (*C*) CPAP failure, resolved with Winx + Provent, in the same patient as in *A* and *B*. As a final step Provent was added, with complete resolution of sleep apnea and sleep fragmentation; the treatment cocktail here is acetazolamide, clonazepam, and Winx + Provent.

predominantly REM-dominant obstructive apnea to predominantly NREM-dominant central apnea/periodic breathing after major weight loss.

Nerve Stimulation

There are no data on the effect of hypoglossal nerve stimulation in patients with mixed apnea. Though speculative, it is plausible that acetazolamide could convert a mixed apnea picture to predominantly obstructive, which is then amenable to treatment with stimulation. Residual sleep fragmentation could also benefit from NREM sleep stabilization. Transvenous phrenic nerve stimulation can lower the central apnea index, but more data are required to establish a clinical role.[56] Sleep efficiency in this study of 19 subjects remained unchanged, raising the possibility that improving respiration comes at the cost of inducing arousals, or at least not treating disease well enough to result in improvements in sleep quality.

Maxillomandibular Advancement

Intuitively, maxillomandibular advancement should be reserved for OSA. However, the author's group has treated more than 10 patients with mixed obstructive and central sleep apnea, with the expectation of needing adjunctive therapy with nasal O_2, acetazolamide, or a sedative, singly or in combination, for optimal benefit; this has indeed been the case as regards requiring these alternatives.

Winx/Oral (Negative) Pressure Therapy

This new approach uses a mouthpiece to apply gentle negative intraoral suction that moves the tongue and soft palate anteriorly, opening and stabilizing the airway.[57] As positive pressure is not applied, perhaps there is less hypocapnia induction. There is no reason why Winx (Apnicure, Redwood City, CA) could not be used with, for example, acetazolamide, to provide complementary and synergistic effects on sleep-breathing, or Winx + nasal oxygen, or Winx + Provent, or indeed Winx + dead space. The author has tried all of these options in the sleep laboratory, and they seem to have potential for benefit in individual patients (**Fig. 7**).

Manipulation of Body Position

A subset of central and complex apnea appears to be very position dependent. These patients are irreparable while supine and "angels" when nonsupine. The reasons include upper airway and lung volume effects, the latter perhaps altering plant gain unfavorably when supine. Positional effects in central apnea syndromes have been reported in patients with classic Cheyne-Stokes respiration in the setting of heart failure.[58,59] Sleeping on the side is also an important adjunctive treatment in reducing positive pressure requirements, as it may cause less CO_2 blow-off and respiratory instability.

A second effect of body position is on fluid redistribution from the caudal to cranial parts of the body.[60–64] In those with central apnea the effect is rapid, and associated with increased neck circumference and hypocapnia from increased lung water. Therapeutic manipulation is currently unwieldy, but a wedge pillow or pillows are options.

SUMMARY

Enhanced or dysregulated respiratory chemoreflexes have a profound impact on sleep-breathing and the polygraphic patterns that emerge. There is an increasing array of treatment options, both on-label and off-label, singly or in combination, that can be used to enhance system stability. Three major components need to be adequately phenotyped and targeted: upper airway, respiratory control, and sleep fragmentation/consolidation. Alternative options for treating central sleep apnea syndromes need to be tested in randomized prospective trials to determine their optimal roles in disease management. Until then, case-by-case trials of effectiveness will be required.

REFERENCES

1. Berry RB, Budhiraja R, Gottlieb DJ, et al. Rules for scoring respiratory events in sleep: update of the 2007 AASM Manual for the Scoring of Sleep and Associated Events. Deliberations of the Sleep Apnea Definitions Task Force of the American Academy of Sleep Medicine. J Clin Sleep Med 2012;8: 597–619.
2. Jobin V, Rigau J, Beauregard J, et al. Evaluation of upper airway patency during Cheyne-Stokes breathing in heart failure patients. Eur Respir J 2012;40:1523–30.
3. Thomas RJ, Tamisier R, Boucher J, et al. Nocturnal hypoxia exposure with simulated altitude for 14 days does not significantly alter working memory or vigilance in humans. Sleep 2007;30:1195–203.
4. Badr MS, Toiber F, Skatrud JB, et al. Pharyngeal narrowing/occlusion during central sleep apnea. J Appl Physiol 1995;78:1806–15.
5. Sankri-Tarbichi AG, Rowley JA, Badr MS. Expiratory pharyngeal narrowing during central

hypocapnic hypopnea. Am J Respir Crit Care Med 2009;179:313–9.

6. Westhoff M, Arzt M, Litterst P. Prevalence and treatment of central sleep apnoea emerging after initiation of continuous positive airway pressure in patients with obstructive sleep apnoea without evidence of heart failure. Sleep Breath 2012;16:71–8.

7. Javaheri S, Smith J, Chung E. The prevalence and natural history of complex sleep apnea. J Clin Sleep Med 2009;5:205–11.

8. Thomas RJ, Terzano MG, Parrino L, et al. Obstructive sleep-disordered breathing with a dominant cyclic alternating pattern—a recognizable polysomnographic variant with practical clinical implications. Sleep 2004;27:229–34.

9. Thomas RJ, Mietus JE, Peng CK, et al. Differentiating obstructive from central and complex sleep apnea using an automated electrocardiogram-based method. Sleep 2007;30:1756–69.

10. Xie A, Bedekar A, Skatrud JB, et al. The heterogeneity of obstructive sleep apnea (predominant obstructive vs pure obstructive apnea). Sleep 2011;34:745–50.

11. Loewen A, Ostrowski M, Laprairie J, et al. Determinants of ventilatory instability in obstructive sleep apnea: inherent or acquired? Sleep 2009;32:1355–65.

12. Meza S, Mendez M, Ostrowski M, et al. Susceptibility to periodic breathing with assisted ventilation during sleep in normal subjects. J Appl Physiol 1998;85:1929–40.

13. Younes M. Role of respiratory control mechanisms in the pathogenesis of obstructive sleep disorders. J Appl Physiol 2008;105:1389–405.

14. Younes M, Ostrowski M, Atkar R, et al. Mechanisms of breathing instability in patients with obstructive sleep apnea. J Appl Physiol 2007;103:1929–41.

15. Younes M, Ostrowski M, Thompson W, et al. Chemical control stability in patients with obstructive sleep apnea. Am J Respir Crit Care Med 2001;163:1181–90.

16. Thomas RJ. Strong chemoreflex modulation of sleep-breathing: some answers but even more questions. J Clin Sleep Med 2009;5:212–4.

17. Wellman A, Edwards BA, Sands SA, et al. A simplified method for determining phenotypic traits in patients with obstructive sleep apnea. J Appl Physiol 2013;114:911–22.

18. Eckert DJ, White DP, Jordan AS, et al. Defining phenotypic causes of obstructive sleep apnea: identification of novel therapeutic targets. Am J Respir Crit Care Med 2013;188(8):996–1004.

19. Szollosi I, Jones M, Morrell MJ, et al. Effect of CO_2 inhalation on central sleep apnea and arousals from sleep. Respiration 2004;71:493–8.

20. Khayat RN, Xie A, Patel AK, et al. Cardiorespiratory effects of added dead space in patients with heart failure and central sleep apnea. Chest 2003;123:1551–60.

21. Xie A, Teodorescu M, Pegelow DF, et al. Effects of stabilizing or increasing respiratory motor outputs on obstructive sleep apnea. J Appl Physiol 2013;115:22–33.

22. Gilmartin G, McGeehan B, Vigneault K, et al. Treatment of positive airway pressure treatment-associated respiratory instability with enhanced expiratory rebreathing space (EERS). J Clin Sleep Med 2010;6:529–38.

23. Thomas RJ, Daly RW, Weiss JW. Low-concentration carbon dioxide is an effective adjunct to positive airway pressure in the treatment of refractory mixed central and obstructive sleep-disordered breathing. Sleep 2005;28:69–77.

24. Giannoni A, Baruah R, Willson K, et al. Real-time dynamic carbon dioxide administration: a novel treatment strategy for stabilization of periodic breathing with potential application to central sleep apnea. J Am Coll Cardiol 2010;56:1832–7.

25. Sakakibara M, Sakata Y, Usui K, et al. Effectiveness of short-term treatment with nocturnal oxygen therapy for central sleep apnea in patients with congestive heart failure. J Cardiol 2005;46:53–61.

26. Gold AR, Bleecker ER, Smith PL. A shift from central and mixed sleep apnea to obstructive sleep apnea resulting from low-flow oxygen. Am Rev Respir Dis 1985;132:220–3.

27. Allam JS, Olson EJ, Gay PC, et al. Efficacy of adaptive servoventilation in treatment of complex and central sleep apnea syndromes. Chest 2007;132:1839–46.

28. Chowdhuri S, Ghabsha A, Sinha P, et al. Treatment of central sleep apnea in U.S. veterans. J Clin Sleep Med 2012;8:555–63.

29. Parrino L, Ferri R, Bruni O, et al. Cyclic alternating pattern (CAP): the marker of sleep instability. Sleep Med Rev 2012;16:27–45.

30. Thomas RJ, Mietus JE, Peng CK, et al. An electrocardiogram-based technique to assess cardiopulmonary coupling during sleep. Sleep 2005;28:1151–61.

31. Eckert DJ, Owens RL, Kehlmann GB, et al. Eszopiclone increases the respiratory arousal threshold and lowers the apnoea/hypopnoea index in obstructive sleep apnoea patients with a low arousal threshold. Clin Sci (Lond) 2011;120:505–14.

32. Quadri S, Drake C, Hudgel DW. Improvement of idiopathic central sleep apnea with zolpidem. J Clin Sleep Med 2009;5:122–9.

33. Bonnet MH, Dexter JR, Arand DL. The effect of triazolam on arousal and respiration in central sleep apnea patients. Sleep 1990;13:31–41.

34. Guilleminault C, Crowe C, Quera-Salva MA, et al. Periodic leg movement, sleep fragmentation and

central sleep apnoea in two cases: reduction with clonazepam. Eur Respir J 1988;1:762–5.

35. Nickol AH, Leverment J, Richards P, et al. Temazepam at high altitude reduces periodic breathing without impairing next-day performance: a randomized cross-over double-blind study. J Sleep Res 2006;15:445–54.

36. Wang D, Teichtahl H, Drummer O, et al. Central sleep apnea in stable methadone maintenance treatment patients. Chest 2005;128:1348–56.

37. Sharkey KM, Kurth ME, Anderson BJ, et al. Obstructive sleep apnea is more common than central sleep apnea in methadone maintenance patients with subjective sleep complaints. Drug Alcohol Depend 2010;108:77–83.

38. Charpentier A, Bisac S, Poirot I, et al. Sleep quality and apnea in stable methadone maintenance treatment. Subst Use Misuse 2010;45:1431–4.

39. Walker JM, Farney RJ, Rhondeau SM, et al. Chronic opioid use is a risk factor for the development of central sleep apnea and ataxic breathing. J Clin Sleep Med 2007;3:455–61.

40. Teichtahl H, Wang D, Cunnington D, et al. Ventilatory responses to hypoxia and hypercapnia in stable methadone maintenance treatment patients. Chest 2005;128:1339–47.

41. Shore ET, Millman RP. Central sleep apnea and acetazolamide therapy. Arch Intern Med 1983; 143:1278–80.

42. Inoue Y, Takata K, Sakamoto I, et al. Clinical efficacy and indication of acetazolamide treatment on sleep apnea syndrome. Psychiatry Clin Neurosci 1999;53:321–2.

43. Edwards BA, Sands SA, Eckert DJ, et al. Acetazolamide improves loop gain but not the other physiological traits causing obstructive sleep apnoea. J Appl Physiol 2012;590:1199–211.

44. Edwards BA, Connolly JG, Campana LM, et al. Acetazolamide attenuates the ventilatory response to arousal in patients with obstructive sleep apnea. Sleep 2013;36:281–5.

45. Nakayama H, Smith CA, Rodman JR, et al. Effect of ventilatory drive on carbon dioxide sensitivity below eupnea during sleep. Am J Respir Crit Care Med 2002;165:1251–60.

46. Javaheri S. Acetazolamide improves central sleep apnea in heart failure: a double-blind, prospective study. Am J Respir Crit Care Med 2006; 173:234–7.

47. Latshang TD, Nussbaumer-Ochsner Y, Henn RM, et al. Effect of acetazolamide and autoCPAP therapy on breathing disturbances among patients with obstructive sleep apnea syndrome who travel to altitude: a randomized controlled trial. J Am Med Assoc 2012;308:2390–8.

48. Glidewell RN, Orr WC, Imes N. Acetazolamide as an adjunct to CPAP treatment: a case of complex sleep apnea in a patient on long-acting opioid therapy. J Clin Sleep Med 2009;5:63–4.

49. De Simone G, Di Fiore A, Menchise V, et al. Carbonic anhydrase inhibitors. Zonisamide is an effective inhibitor of the cytosolic isozyme II and mitochondrial isozyme V: solution and X-ray crystallographic studies. Bioorg Med Chem Lett 2005; 15:2315–20.

50. Westwood AJ, Vendrame M, Montouris G, et al. Pearls & Oy-sters: treatment of central sleep apnea with topiramate. Neurology 2012;78: e97–9.

51. Sankri-Tarbichi AG, Grullon K, Badr MS. Effects of clonidine on breathing during sleep and susceptibility to central apnoea. Respir Physiol Neurobiol 2013;185:356–61.

52. Patel AV, Hwang D, Masdeu MJ, et al. Predictors of response to a nasal expiratory resistor device and its potential mechanisms of action for treatment of obstructive sleep apnea. J Clin Sleep Med 2011; 7:13–22.

53. Avidan AY. The development of central sleep apnea with an oral appliance. Sleep Med 2006;7: 85–6.

54. Denbar MA. A case study involving the combination treatment of an oral appliance and auto-titrating CPAP unit. Sleep Breath 2002;6: 125–8.

55. El-Solh AA, Moitheennazima B, Akinnusi ME, et al. Combined oral appliance and positive airway pressure therapy for obstructive sleep apnea: a pilot study. Sleep Breath 2011;15:203–8.

56. Zhang XL, Ding N, Wang H, et al. Transvenous phrenic nerve stimulation in patients with Cheyne-Stokes respiration and congestive heart failure: a safety and proof-of-concept study. Chest 2012; 142:927–34.

57. Colrain IM, Black J, Siegel LC, et al. A multicenter evaluation of oral pressure therapy for the treatment of obstructive sleep apnea. Sleep Med 2013;14:830–7.

58. Szollosi I, Roebuck T, Thompson B, et al. Lateral sleeping position reduces severity of central sleep apnea/Cheyne-Stokes respiration. Sleep 2006;29: 1045–51.

59. Joho S, Oda Y, Hirai T, et al. Impact of sleeping position on central sleep apnea/Cheyne-Stokes respiration in patients with heart failure. Sleep Med 2010;11:143–8.

60. White LH, Bradley TD. Role of nocturnal rostral fluid shift in the pathogenesis of obstructive and central sleep apnoea. J Physiol 2013;591:1179–93.

61. Redolfi S, Yumino D, Ruttanaumpawan P, et al. Relationship between overnight rostral fluid shift and obstructive sleep apnea in nonobese men. Am J Respir Crit Care Med 2009;179: 241–6.

62. Kasai T, Motwani SS, Yumino D, et al. Differing relationship of nocturnal fluid shifts to sleep apnea in men and women with heart failure. Circ Heart Fail 2012;5:467–74.

63. Friedman O, Bradley TD, Chan CT, et al. Relationship between overnight rostral fluid shift and obstructive sleep apnea in drug-resistant hypertension. Hypertension 2010;56:1077–82.

64. Elias RM, Bradley TD, Kasai T, et al. Rostral overnight fluid shift in end-stage renal disease: relationship with obstructive sleep apnea. Nephrol Dial Transplant 2012;27:1569–73.

Central Hypoventilation Syndromes

Christopher M. Cielo, DO[a], Carole L. Marcus, MBBCh[b],*

KEYWORDS

- Central hypoventilation • CCHS • PHOX2B • ROHHAD • Autonomic dysfunction • Children
- Home ventilation • Noninvasive ventilation

KEY POINTS

- Ventilation is a complex, tightly regulated process involving voluntary and involuntary responses to changes in pH, oxygenation, and Pco_2.
- Congenital central hypoventilation syndrome is caused by a defect in the *PHOX2B* gene and has distinct phenotypic findings.
- Rapid-onset obesity with hypothalamic dysfunction, hypoventilation, and autonomic dysregulation is characterized by rapid weight gain and hypoventilation without any mutation in *PHOX2B*.
- There is significant variability in the degree of hypoventilation across conditions, but hypoventilation is worse during sleep in all conditions.
- Mechanical ventilation is the mainstay of therapy for central alveolar hypoventilation, but a multidisciplinary team is often required to manage these complex conditions.

INTRODUCTION

Hypoventilation refers to an increased arterial concentration of serum carbon dioxide due to inadequate gas exchange. Central hypoventilation indicates that a deficiency in the central nervous system, rather than the respiratory system, is the root of the problem. Central hypoventilation is uncommon and may be due to a variety of conditions (**Table 1**), which can be either congenital or acquired. The following is a review of conditions causing central hypoventilation in children. Although individually rare, these conditions can have serious effects on children if not identified, and understanding the pathophysiology of these conditions will help direct management and provide optimal care.

NORMAL CONTROL OF BREATHING

Control of breathing is governed by a complex system of receptors responding to changes in Po_2, Pco_2, and pH, as well as other factors, such as lung stretch, that has significant redundancy and changes with age and sleep state. Central chemoreceptors, located in multiple areas of the brainstem, respond to small changes in Pco_2, causing stimulation of breathing by the central pattern generator in response to hypercapnia.[1] Central chemoreceptors are thought to be responsible for more than 50% of the hypercapnic ventilatory response. Peripheral chemoreceptors, located at the bifurcation of the carotid arteries, respond to acidemia, transient hypercapnia, or low Po_2 in arterial blood.[2] The central chemoreceptors account

Disclosures: Dr C.L. Marcus has received research support from Philips Respironics and Ventus, not related to the current article.

a Division of Pulmonary Medicine, The Children's Hospital of Philadelphia, Colket Translational Research Building, 11th Floor Pulmonary Medicine, 3501 Civic Center Boulevard, Philadelphia, PA 19104, USA; b Department of Pediatrics, Sleep Center, The Children's Hospital of Philadelphia, The University of Pennsylvania Perelman School of Medicine, 9 Northwest 50 Main Building, 34th and Civic Center Boulevard, Philadelphia, PA 19104, USA

* Corresponding author.

E-mail address: marcus@email.chop.edu

Table 1
Summary of central hypoventilation syndromes in childhood

Syndrome	Diagnosis/Unique Clinical Features	Age of Onset	Treatment/Prognosis
CCHS	*PHOX2B* mutation necessary for diagnosis Associated with Hirschsprung disease, neural crest tumors, arrhythmias	Usually at birth	All will require assisted ventilation; diaphragmatic pacing an option for some with 24-h ventilatory needs Good overall prognosis with adequate care but will require ongoing ventilatory support
ROHHAD	No diagnostic test Associated with rapid weight gain, growth hormone deficiency, developmental delay, behavioral problems	Variable after 1.5 y old; symptoms may appear years apart	All will require ventilation; significant neurologic and psychiatric morbidity in some patients
FD	Caused by mutations in I-K-B complex protein Associated with blood pressure instability, temperature instability, ataxia, dysphagia, renal disease	Symptoms present at birth	Supportive therapy: some will benefit from ventilation, may require feeding tube, renal/cardiac evaluation
Chiari malformation	Diagnosis by magnetic resonance imaging CM II associated with myelomeningocele	Usually at birth; milder cases may present later	Posterior fossa decompression successful in treating central apnea in some patients; some will require ventilation, often noninvasive
PWS	Caused by gene deletion at 15q11–13 Patients present with infantile hypotonia and failure to thrive followed by hyperphagia, morbid obesity, developmental delay, and behavior problems	Usually infancy	High risk for obstructive sleep apnea and other sleep disorders; some will require ventilation, usually noninvasive Monitor closely for sleep-disordered breathing after starting growth hormone; significant psychosocial morbidity
Achondroplasia	Caused by mutation in fibroblast growth factor 3 Associated with short limbs with brachydactyly, hypotonia	Usually infancy	Nocturnal hypoxemia is common If hypoventilation or central apnea present, obtain imaging to evaluate for impingement at foramen magnum Overall good prognosis
Mitochondrial disorders	Group of rare disorders affecting mitochondria metabolism Focal necrotizing lesions seen on brain imaging Associated with progressive psychomotor decline	Usually first few months of life	Some will benefit from ventilatory support No specific therapies Poor prognosis

for greater than half of the ventilatory response to CO_2 with the peripheral chemoreceptors contributing the remainder of the response.[3] The retrotrapezoid nucleus, a sparsely populated collection of neurons at the ventral medullary surface, is an important source of respiratory drive. The neurons in this nucleus are sensitive to changes in both oxygenation and ventilation as it receives input from the carotid bodies, hypothalamus, J receptors, and central pattern generator. The retrotrapezoid nucleus is hypothesized to be the intrinsic respiratory pacemaker at birth.[4] The medullary raphe is another central nervous system site potentially responsive to CO_2 changes.

To a degree, the brainstem centers of metabolic control of breathing can be overridden by anatomically distinct centers, which allow for voluntary control of breathing, thus allowing actions such as hyperventilation and breath-holding. In normal individuals, awareness of breathing increases with increased respiratory load, exercise, and upper airway obstruction, and voluntary control is affected by emotions such as laughter or panic. Although metabolic control of breathing is located in the brainstem, voluntary control of breathing is anatomically located in the cerebellum, primary motor cortex, and premotor areas.[1] Final integration of the voluntary and metabolic centers of respiratory control is thought to be located in the spinal motor neurons or the brainstem. The stimuli to the brainstem resulting in the feeling of dyspnea originate from vagal afferents.

In normal individuals, CO_2 tension is the primary trigger for ventilation. Above an apneic threshold, the ventilatory response to CO_2 is linear and is affected by sleep state and hypoxemia.[2] In response to increasing P_{CO_2}, ventilation will initially increase by greater tidal volume, followed by an increase in respiratory rate. In response to hypoxia, ventilation initially increases but then is reduced over time. In infants, this ventilatory "roll-off" will reach a reduction in ventilation that is below normoxic breathing in the second part of this biphasic response. In older children and adults, however, there is a more modest decline in ventilation after the ventilatory peak in response to hypoxia.[5] The ventilatory response to combined hypoxia and hypercapnia is multiplicative rather than additive.

At the initiation of sleep, upper airway resistance increases, but withdrawal of the wakefulness stimulus leads to an immediate increase in CO_2, which is not due entirely to changes in pulmonary mechanics.[6] During rapid eye movement (REM) sleep, there is often a further increase in CO_2 due to loss of accessory ventilatory muscle tone. The presence of sleep also causes the emergence of the apneic threshold, which is overridden by cortical influences during wakefulness. In individuals where there is a narrow gap between eupnic and apneic CO_2 levels, such as infants, unstable breathing patterns such as periodic breathing may emerge. In addition, the ventilatory responses to hypercapnia and hypoxemia are blunted during sleep. During REM sleep, there is less input from brainstem centers and more input from the primary motor cortex, resulting in more variation in the respiratory pattern.[7] Arousal is an important response to changes in oxygenation or ventilation during sleep. Although hypoxemia is a strong stimulus for arousal in the first few months of life, elevated carbon dioxide levels are the more robust stimuli for arousal in later life.[8]

CONGENITAL CENTRAL HYPOVENTILATION SYNDROME
Background and Genetics

Congenital central hypoventilation syndrome (CCHS) is a rare, lifelong condition that causes primary alveolar hypoventilation. First described in 1970 by Mellins and colleagues,[9] it was discovered in 2003 that the paired-like homeobox 2B (PHOX2B) gene on chromosome 4p12 is the disease-defining gene for CCHS.[10,11] Transmission is through an autosomal-dominant pattern, although most cases of CCHS are de novo or inherited from a mosaic typically unaffected parent.[10,11] PHOX2B encodes a transcription factor that is instrumental in the regulation of neural crest migration and development of the autonomic nervous system. More than 90% of patients with CCHS are heterozygous for an in-frame polyalanine repeat of the 20-residue polyalanine region. Although the normal genotype is referred to as 20/20, these mutated proteins produce genotypes of 20/24 to 20/33. The remaining approximately 10% of PHOX2B mutations are nonpolyalanine repeat mutations (NPARMs) causing missense, nonsense, or frameshifts.[12] The incidence of CCHS is currently unknown, but one French study has estimated a rate of 1 in 200,000 live births.[13]

Clinical Presentation

Children with CCHS usually present during infancy with episodes of cyanosis or apnea, or even cardiorespiratory arrest. Characteristically, children with CCHS have been described as having a square face with a tall, flat forehead, and a deep philtrum with downturned lips.[14] This phenotype is more prevalent with increased polyalanine repeats. There may be ophthalmologic clues to a diagnosis of CCHS as well. Children with CCHS may have a sluggish to absent papillary light reflex, strabismus, anisocoria, or convergence insufficiency. Individuals presenting late in the course may have evidence of right heart failure or developmental delay.

Some children will present outside of infancy and even in adulthood, but a careful history will often reveal signs and symptoms of hypoventilation or disorders of autonomic regulation from the newborn period. Those not diagnosed until much later may present with the sequelae of longstanding hypoventilation and hypoxemia, including epilepsy or cognitive disabilities.[12] CCHS should also be considered in older individuals with hypoventilation associated with respiratory infections or anesthesia. CCHS diagnosed in children over 1 month of age is termed later-onset CCHS. These children usually have the 20/24 and 20/25 genotypes and rarely have NPARMs.

The degree of hypoventilation in patients with CCHS is variable, and although most children ventilate adequately during wakefulness, approximately 15% require ventilatory support even when awake. Typically, a greater number of polyalanine repeats correlate with more severe hypoventilation, with those having 20/27 and 20/33 genotypes often requiring ventilatory support during both sleep and wakefulness. Because individuals with CCHS lack the response to hypercapnia and hypoxemia, they do not adequately augment respiratory effort required during ventilatory challenges such as illness or exercise. One study found that during an exercise challenge, children with CCHS, who had absent hypercapnic and hypoxic ventilatory responses during wakefulness, increased minute ventilation by increasing respiratory rate but not tidal volume.[15] Interestingly, this study showed a positive correlation between treadmill pace and respiratory rate. Oxygen saturation decreased and CO_2 tension increased during exercise in patients with CCHS but not controls in this study. A different study of 6 sleeping patients with CCHS demonstrated increased respiratory rate during brief periods of passive lower extremity motion.[16] These studies suggest that mechanoreceptors in the limbs play a role in regulating ventilation in children with CCHS.

The pathophysiology associated with hypoventilation from CCHS is not well understood. Multiple studies have evaluated central and peripheral chemoreceptor function in children with CCHS. Patients with CCHS have been shown to have a peripheral chemoreceptor response similar to controls when given rapid challenges of hyperoxic or hypercarbic gas, suggesting that peripheral chemoreceptors are present and functioning in patients with CCHS who can ventilate adequately when awake.[17] However, classic rebreathing responses to longer hypoxic or hypercapnic challenges are abnormal.[18] One study evaluating respiratory-related evoked potentials found disrupted central integration of the afferent signal during wakefulness and reduced responses during non-REM sleep in patients with central hypoventilation syndrome compared with controls.[19] Another study found that, compared with controls, patients with CCHS had no difference in cough threshold when evoked by fog inhalation, but those with CCHS lacked respiratory sensations or increases in ventilation before coughing.[20] Functional magnetic resonance imaging has also been used to evaluate central nervous system signal responses in the brains of people with CCHS. Compared with controls, delayed responses have been demonstrated in the medullary sensory regions, limbic areas, and cerebellar and pontine sensorimotor coordination areas in patients with CCHS during Valsalva.[21,22] Functional magnetic resonance imaging studies evaluating response to hyperoxia have shown altered responses in the amygdala, which normally regulates respiratory timing, as well as blunted heart rate responses in patients with CCHS compared with controls.[23] This combination of findings underlies the autonomic dysfunction central to CCHS and supports the hypothesis that deficiencies in central integration of chemoreceptor inputs, rather than the receptors themselves, are likely responsible for the autonomic dysfunction and loss of respiratory drive in CCHS.

Sleep Findings

During sleep, infants with CCHS usually have reduced tidal volumes with regular respiration and periods of central apnea. Hypoventilation is present during wakefulness but is more profound during sleep (**Fig. 1**). A study of 9 children breathing spontaneously during sleep found more pronounced hypoventilation during non-REM than REM sleep, although significant hypoventilation was seen in all sleep stages.[19] The cause of this state dependency is unknown, but may be related to a REM-related ventilatory drive not yet well understood. However, ventilatory support is required throughout all sleep stages.

Associated Conditions

A variety of other autonomic nervous system dysregulations has been associated with CCHS, including Hirschsprung disease in about 20% of patients and neural crest tumors, which are usually in individuals with NPARMs.[12] Other symptoms of autonomic dysfunction, including temperature instability, cardiac arrhythmias that may require a pacemaker, reduced pupillary light response,

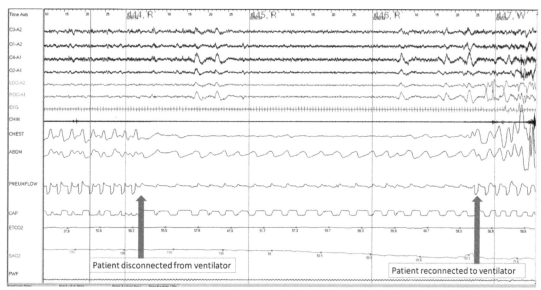

Fig. 1. One hundred twenty-second polysomnogram epoch of a mechanically ventilated 20-year-old patient with CCHS, 20/26 genotype. When briefly disconnected from the ventilator, there is a dramatic decrease in airflow and the patient desaturates to 77% and $ETCO_2$ increases by 10 mm Hg. Y-axis parameters: time axis, clock time (in s) with the epoch number superimposed; C3-A2, O1-A2, C4-A1, and O2-A1 are EEG leads; LOC-A2 and ROC-A1 are left and right electrooculograms, respectively. ABDM, abdominal wall motion; CAP, end-tidal P_{CO_2} waveform; CHEST, chest wall motion; CHIN, submental EMG signal; $ETCO_2$, end-tidal P_{CO_2} value; PNEUMOFLOW, airflow measured with a pneumotachograph; PWF, oximeter pulse waveform; SAO_2, arterial oxygen saturation.

esophageal dysmotility, and abnormal perception of discomfort or anxiety, are also seen.[12,24]

Diagnostic Evaluation

A diagnosis of CCHS should be considered in any child who has hypoventilation without known dysfunction of the brainstem, neuromuscular weakness, cardiopulmonary, or metabolic cause to explain the finding. A 2-stage blood test is available for the diagnosis of CCHS and should be sent in any case where the diagnosis is considered. The *PHOX2B* Screening Test, which is a gel electrophoresis that evaluates for the polyalanine repeat mutations and the most common NPARMs, is capable of identifying 95% of CCHS cases. If this test is negative and the phenotype supports the diagnosis, the *PHOX2B* Sequencing Test can be performed.[12] Hemoglobin and hematocrit for polycythemia and blood gas with bicarbonate level should be considered to evaluate for respiratory acidosis and metabolic alkalosis as ongoing evaluations. Echocardiogram, electrocardiogram, and brain-type natriuretic peptide levels should be considered annually to evaluate for pulmonary hypertension.

Polysomnography is extremely useful in the evaluation of CCHS. This study should include evaluation of wakefulness, REM, and non-REM sleep to assess the degree of hypoventilation.

Ventilatory response testing has been used as a research tool to assess the patient's ventilatory responses to both hypercapnia and hypoxia.

The differential diagnosis is broad and includes primary pulmonary, cardiac, neurologic, or metabolic disease. To evaluate for underlying lung disease, chest imaging with radiography or computed tomography should be considered, as well as pulmonary function testing if possible. Intracranial lesions should be evaluated with magnetic resonance imaging. Inborn errors of metabolism can be evaluated with metabolic testing and potentially muscle biopsy.

Management of CCHS

All patients with CCHS require mechanical ventilation; therapy with oxygen or respiratory stimulants is not adequate. Infants may require continuous ventilation because of an immature respiratory system and circadian rhythm. Many infants will require tracheostomy to achieve adequate ventilation, but older children may be able to be ventilated with noninvasive ventilation (see Management of central hypoventilation syndromes section). CCHS is a lifelong condition and although the ventilatory system will become more stable with age, patients will not develop normal ventilatory responses to hypoxia or hypercarbia. Mortality is highly variable, and the main causes of death are cor pulmonale, pneumonia, and aspiration.[13] With adequate ventilation and well-coordinated care, however, many patients with CCHS can expect to lead productive lives. There is a growing cohort of patients with CCHS surviving to adulthood and even having children of their own. Genetic counseling is important, especially considering the dominant nature of transmission.

RAPID-ONSET OBESITY WITH HYPOTHALAMIC DYSFUNCTION, HYPOVENTILATION AND AUTONOMIC DYSREGULATION

Rapid-onset obesity with hypothalamic dysfunction, hypoventilation and autonomic dysregulation (ROHHAD), also known as late-onset central hypoventilation with hypothalamic dysfunction, is a rare disorder presenting in childhood with rapid weight gain, hypothalamic endocrine dysfunction, and severe hypoventilation. Children often present in crisis, such as respiratory failure or cor pulmonale. This condition was first described in 1965[25] but has only recently been distinguished from CCHS as a separate condition.[26,27] Although CCHS typically presents during infancy, the clinical findings associated with ROHHAD begin after 1.5 years of age, with a mean age of approximately 3 years.[26] Rapid onset of obesity is typically the first clinical sign in ROHHAD and is striking, often with 15 kg or more of weight gain in a single year (**Fig. 2**). Additional hypothalamic dysfunction may precede or follow weight gain and may include growth hormone deficiency, hyperprolactinemia, central hypothyroidism, disordered water balance, precocious/delayed puberty, thermal dysregulation, or corticotrophin deficiency. Because of these important features, children in whom ROHHAD is being considered should be evaluated and followed by an endocrinologist. Developmental delay and regression as well as behavioral problems are also common. Children with ROHHAD are also at risk for neural crest tumors, including ganglioneuromas and ganglioneuroblastomas.[28] Similar to CCHS, ophthalmologic abnormalities may be seen in individuals with ROHHAD.[26]

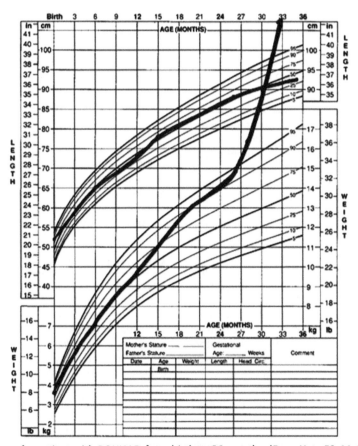

Fig. 2. Growth curve of a patient with ROHHAD from birth to 36 months. (*From* Katz ES, McGrath S, Marcus CL. Late-onset central hypoventilation with hypothalamic dysfunction: a distinct clinical syndrome. Pediatr Pulmonol 2000;29(1):64. Copyright John Wiley & Sons; with permission.)

In addition to hypothalamic dysfunction, children with ROHHAD develop hypoventilation. The respiratory phenotype of ROHHAD includes an absent or attenuated response to hypercarbia and/or hypoxemia and can be evaluated with hypercapnic ventilatory response testing. In one of the largest series reported, about half of patients with ROHHAD required tracheostomy for positive pressure ventilation.[26]

Unlike CCHS, mutations of PHOX2B are characteristically lacking from individuals with ROHHAD.[29] To date, no candidate genes have been identified as a cause of ROHHAD[30] and studies continue to attempt to identify the presumed genetic basis of ROHHAD.

The prognosis of ROHHAD has improved with earlier identification and treatment of the condition. Significant morbidity exists from a progressive neurologic or psychiatric decline in a subset of cases, including seizures, depression, psychosis, hallucinations, and emotional lability. Autonomic nervous system dysregulation can cause severe bradycardia in some patients. The care of individuals is complex and should be multidisciplinary, focus on the endocrine and ventilatory abnormalities, and include assisted ventilation when hypoventilation occurs.

FAMILIAL DYSAUTONOMIA

Familial dysautonomia (FD) is a rare autosomal-recessive condition primarily affecting the Ashkenazi Jewish population, that was first described in 1949.[31] FD is caused by mutations in the gene that encodes for I-K-B complex associated protein, affecting the development of primary sensory neurons. As a result, people with FD have severe blood pressure instability, impairment in temperature perception, sense of taste, and ability to swallow, as well as ataxia.[32] Individuals with FD are prone to developmental abnormalities, renal disease, and left ventricular hypertrophy, in addition to vomiting attacks from surges in sympathetic activity.[33,34]

Patients with FD have been shown to have abnormal ventilatory responses to hypoxia and hypercapnia. One study of 22 subjects with FD showed that progressive hypoxia resulted in blunted increases in ventilation and paradoxic decreases in heart rate and blood pressure. Hyperventilation induced prolonged apneas with profound desaturations.[35] A study using inductance plethysmography and electrocardiogram at home in 25 children with FD found an increased respiratory frequency and greater daytime respiratory variability in those with FD compared with controls.[36] Children with FD have more apnea and desaturation than controls during sleep.[37]

There is no definitive therapy for FD and treatment is supportive, but early recognition of FD is related to better survival rates.[38] Because of swallowing difficulty, chronic lung disease secondary to chronic aspiration is a concern in young children. Gastrostomy tube and/or fundoplication should be considered.[39] Because of associated autonomic neuropathy, there are a host of potential surgical complications involving the respiratory, cardiovascular, and renal systems. Perioperatively, adequate pain control is important to prevent crises from sympathetic surges.[40] Pulmonary causes of death are common, frequently during sleep. Sudden unexplained deaths are reported in nearly a third of cases.[38]

CHIARI MALFORMATION

In a Chiari type II malformation (CM II), the cerebellar vermis, caudal brain stem, and fourth ventricle herniate through the foramen magnum, obstructing flow of cerebrospinal fluid and causing hydrocephalus. This type of malformation is usually associated with myelomeningocele, where the meninges and spinal cord protrude through open vertebral arches leading to paralysis and significant morbidity and mortality.[41]

Individuals with myelomeningocele and CM II have blunted ventilatory response to hypercapnia and hypoxemia, which suggests abnormalities of central chemoreceptors. In a study of 7 infants with myelomeningocele and Chiari malformation, arousal to hypercapnia occurred in only 37.5% of subjects compared with 100% of controls. Arousal to hypoxia was also diminished, with only 18.2% of those with myelomeningocele arousing compared with 89% of controls.[42] The cause of central hypoventilation in patients with Chiari malformation is thought to be due to dysgenesis of neural structures or damage to the brainstem and cerebellum during the herniation, causing impairment of the respiratory centers.[43]

Individuals with CM II are also at risk for sleep-disordered breathing. In a population-based study of 73 children, 16% had central hypoventilation, but 41% and 27% had obstructive and central apnea, respectively.[44] This study also reported several children who had sleep-related hypoxemia not related to apnea or hypoventilation. A recent study of 16 children with CM II reported a relatively high mean central apnea index of 5.9 ± 7.3 events/h, but this study did not report CO_2 measurements.[45] Individuals with myelomeningocele have also been shown to have a high rate of restrictive lung disease and many have respiratory muscle weakness.[46]

Children with CM II have variable presentation, with the most severely affected patients presenting in infancy with apnea, bradycardia, and vocal cord paralysis.[47] Children with meningomyelocele should be evaluated with a polysomnogram that includes CO_2 monitoring. If abnormalities are seen, an evaluation of hydrocephalus should be made. If abnormalities persist despite correction of hydrocephalus, cervical decompression may be considered. However, the abnormalities may be secondary to dysplasia of the brainstem rather than compression and may not resolve after surgery.[44] Some children with CM II, particularly those with myelomeningocele and without spontaneous ventilation in infancy, will require mechanical ventilation, as there is an increased mortality in this population due to hypoventilation and central apnea.

There is no definitive evidence to suggest that Chiari type I (CM I) malformation is related to hypoventilation, but there are reports of significant sleep-disordered breathing in patients with CM I malformations. One case report documents a young man with a CM I with syringomyelia who presented with obstructive sleep apnea and hypoventilation after acute respiratory failure. The patient underwent posterior fossa decompression and had improvement in arterial Pco_2 during wakefulness from 65 to 45 mm Hg but his severe obstructive sleep apnea did not improve.[48] There are several reports of children with CM I having significant bradypnea and central apnea.[49,50] Other reports have identified mixed obstructive and central apneas.[51,52] Posterior fossa decompression has been successful in some reports, but there is no large series evaluating ventilation during sleep in CM I.

Prader-Willi Syndrome

Prader-Willi syndrome (PWS) is a condition caused by a deletion of paternally expressed imprinted genes at chromosome 15q11–q13 that results in a phenotype including infantile hypotonia and failure to thrive. As children get older, they develop hyperphagia and obesity as well as developmental delay and behavioral problems.[53] Craniofacial features include a narrow nasal bridge and micrognathia.

Patients with PWS have been shown to have an abnormal ventilatory response. Although eucapnic at rest during wakefulness, individuals with PWS have been shown to have a paradoxic response to hyperoxia and no change in minute ventilation in response to hypercapnia.[54] Obese patients

with PWS have a flattened slope of the ventilatory response curve, but both lean and obese people with PWS begin to increase ventilation at a higher Pco_2 than controls.[55] During sleep, children with PWS have a higher arousal threshold to hypercapnia than control.[56] In response to hypoxia during sleep, people with PWS are less likely to arouse and have a blunted increase in heart rate and respiratory rate compared with controls.[57] These findings suggest abnormal function of both peripheral and central chemoreceptors.

Children with PWS are at risk for a variety of sleep disorders, including altered sleep architecture and both central and obstructive sleep apnea.[58] Obstructive sleep apnea and obstructive hypoventilation may be due to unique features of PWS, including morbid obesity, a small nasopharynx, and hypopharyngeal hypotonia. Young children with PWS may be at risk for developing worsening of sleep-disordered breathing soon after the initiation of growth hormone[59] and there have been reports of sudden death in this population,[60,61] so children with PWS should have a polysomnogram to screen for sleep-disordered breathing before starting therapy.[62] After initiating growth hormone, patients should be closely monitored for signs of sleep-disordered breathing and repeat polysomnography should be considered.

Achondroplasia

Achondroplasia is an autosomal-dominant condition caused by a mutation in the gene encoding fibroblast growth factor receptor type 3 and affects longitudinal growth and craniofacial, vertebral, and neurologic development. Clinical characteristics include mid face hypoplasia, hypotonia, lumbar spinal stenosis, and characteristic short limbs with short, broad fingers (brachydactyly). There may be contraction of the base of the skull with a small foramen magnum.[63,64]

Patients with achondroplasia are at risk for a variety of respiratory conditions. One study of 88 children with achondroplasia found that 47% had abnormal polysomnograms, with hypoxemia being the most common finding, which may be related to mild restrictive lung disease due to a relatively small thorax.[65] A smaller number of patients have obstructive or central apnea, although there is significant variability between studies and prevalence is difficult to estimate.[66]

Disproportion between the size of the skull and its base puts these children at risk for compression of the spinal cord or brainstem at the foramen magnum. This complication of achondroplasia has been implicated in more significant respiratory complications, including sudden death due to apnea in infancy[67] as well as hypoventilation, which can be severe.[68,69] Any child with achondroplasia who has hypoventilation or central apnea should have imaging of the brain and spinal cord to evaluate for impingement. If present, cervicomedullary decompression may be required.[70]

Mitochondrial Disorders

Disorders affecting mitochondrial metabolism may also result in central hypoventilation. Leigh syndrome, also known as subacute necrotizing encephalopathy, first described in 1951, is a rare, progressive neurodegenerative disorder marked by functional brainstem decline. This condition is now recognized to be a group of disorders marked by focal, necrotizing lesions. Patients are often normal during infancy but present with psychomotor regression, weakness, hypotonia, intention tremor, and lactic acidosis during the first 2 years of life.[71] Respiratory failure is a frequent feature of Leigh syndrome, which may be attributed to involvement of the brainstem or respiratory muscle weakness as the condition progresses. Although there are reports of patients surviving until adulthood, in most cases, the condition causes death by 5 years of age.[71] There is no causal therapy for Leigh syndrome and the benefits of mechanical ventilation must be weighed against the poor prognosis.

Central hypoventilation has been described in other disorders of mitochondrial metabolism, including pyruvate dehydrogenase deficiency, Kearns-Sayre syndrome, ophthalmoplegia plus, and other inherited mitochondrial myopathies.[72–75]

Acquired Conditions Causing Central Hypoventilation

In addition to congenital conditions causing central alveolar hypoventilation, damage to respiratory centers in the brain can produce a similar phenotype in previously healthy children. Conditions causing acquired central hypoventilation include brain tumors, central nervous system infections, encephalitis, trauma, and sequelae from neurosurgical procedures.[76–80] The degree of resultant hypoventilation varies from mild to severe depending on the respiratory centers affected and the degree of damage. Some patients will have intermittent apneic episodes and others will require mechanical ventilation, but most ventilatory abnormalities will worsen during sleep. Hypoventilation should be considered in patients with tumors affecting respiratory control centers or those who have a history of central nervous system malignancies and respiratory disease.

MANAGEMENT OF CENTRAL HYPOVENTILATION SYNDROMES
Ventilatory Support

Positive pressure ventilation
The goal of treatment for all patients with central hypoventilation syndromes is adequate ventilation and oxygenation during both sleep and wakefulness in a way that maintains a high quality of life and maximizes the child's ability to participate in school and recreational activities (**Fig. 3**). The amount of ventilatory assistance required in central hypoventilation syndromes is highly variable. In CCHS, for example, although infants usually require continuous mechanical ventilation, older children often achieve adequate ventilation during wakefulness as the respiratory system and circadian rhythm mature.

Positive pressure ventilation via tracheostomy is the most efficacious mode to ensure adequate ventilation when continuous ventilation is required. Difficulties with this type of ventilation include the requirement for the continuous presence of trained caregivers and the risk of death due to tracheostomy decannulation, infection, and speech delays.[81] Advantages of this method include the

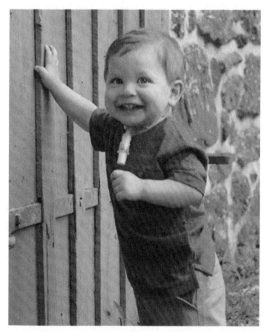

Fig. 3. Sixteen-month-old boy with CCHS. Many children with central hypoventilation syndromes, including those dependent on positive pressure ventilation, can lead happy and fulfilling lives. Note that this child has a tracheostomy tube with flexible tube extension for greater mobility when ventilated and heat moisture exchanger to provide humidification when not connected to a ventilator. (*Courtesy of* Brianne Elizabeth.)

ability to have the patient's face free of a mask and to use a portable, battery-operated ventilator and deliver high pressures if needed.

Noninvasive positive pressure ventilation (NIPPV) allows ventilatory support to be delivered via nasal or face mask, avoids tracheostomy, and is a good option for many children, especially those who require only nocturnal ventilation.[82] Children requiring very high ventilatory pressures, who cannot tolerate or be properly fitted for a mask (such as young infants), or who require continuous ventilation are not good candidates for NIPPV. As with ventilation delivered via tracheostomy, NIPPV settings should be determined and titrated periodically in the sleep laboratory or an intensive care setting. Because many children with central hypoventilation syndromes will not trigger the ventilator adequately during sleep, a mode that provides bilevel pressure at a set rate with a set inspiratory time is preferred.[83]

Negative pressure ventilation

Negative pressure ventilation (NPV) generates a negative inspiratory pressure around the chest and abdomen with a dome-shaped bell, causing inspiration. It was developed to treat respiratory failure during the polio epidemic but there are reports of children with central hypoventilation who have been managed with success using NPV.[84] Children using NPV must remain supine; the units are not portable, and it may be uncomfortable for some people. The use of NPV has been limited by the risk of asynchrony between vocal cord opening and thoracic inspiratory efforts, causing obstructive sleep apnea.[85] NPV is used infrequently now that noninvasive pressure ventilation is available.

Diaphragmatic pacing

Diaphragmatic pacing involves electrical stimulation of the phrenic nerve via a battery-operated external transmitter, generating breathing using the child's own diaphragm as the respiratory pump.[86] Bilateral surgical implantation of phrenic nerve electrodes and diaphragm pacer receivers is recommended in children to achieve optimal ventilation. Pacing is typically initiated 4 to 6 weeks after implantation and requires several months to attain full pacing.[87] These pacers can be used for approximately 12 to 15 hours a day and can offer freedom from a mechanical ventilator during the day. In some cases, older patients may be able to achieve adequate ventilation with the use of a diaphragmatic pacer at night. Complications of diaphragmatic pacers include equipment failure, infection, and fibrosis or tension of the phrenic nerve.[88] Obstructive apnea can occur due to lack of synchronous upper airway skeletal muscle contraction with paced inspiration.[89]

Respiratory stimulants

Although there are case reports of respiratory stimulants treating alveolar hypoventilation,[90] there is no medication that effectively treats central hypoventilation syndromes.

General considerations

Central nervous system depressants such as opiates and benzodiazepines should be avoided when possible. Conditions that cause metabolic alkalosis will decrease respiratory drive and should be aggressively corrected. Increased risk for hypoxia occurs at high altitudes, airplane travel, underwater swimming, and pneumonia, and families should be counseled about the risks of these activities. As children with central hypoventilation are at high risk for respiratory decompensation from respiratory illness, they should get the seasonal influenza vaccine annually. Similar to patients with lung disease, children with central hypoventilation syndromes should avoid exposure to second-hand smoke and be counseled not to smoke themselves. Due to the complexities of these conditions, many children will require psychosocial support.

Anesthesiologists should be aware of the degree of ventilatory requirements for patients with central hypoventilation. Although children with central hypoventilation syndromes can successfully undergo general anesthesia, these children require careful monitoring of gas exchange during and after anesthesia.[91,92] They may require an increase in baseline ventilatory support following the procedure. Anesthetic drugs with the shortest half-life should be chosen and regional anesthesia should be used when possible.[93]

Polysomnography is a useful tool in evaluating hypoxemia and hypoventilation during both wakefulness and sleep and ensuring adequate nocturnal oxygenation and ventilation.[83] Guidelines for CCHS recommend comprehensive respiratory evaluation, including polysomnogram, at least annually,[12] and a similar approach could be taken for other causes of central hypoventilation.

SUMMARY

Conditions causing central alveolar hypoventilation are uncommon in children, but have a profound impact on the lives of those affected. As research continues to elucidate the underlying mechanisms behind these conditions, the goal will be better identification and treatment of respiratory and nonrespiratory manifestations. Current therapy for central hypoventilation focuses on achieving normal gas exchange, primarily through mechanical ventilation. Early identification of central hypoventilation and initiation of appropriate ventilation strategies can help to improve outcomes associated with chronic hypoxemia. As with all complex pediatric medical conditions, the difficulties of different modes of mechanical ventilation must always be weighed against the child's overall quality of life to determine the most appropriate therapy. Many children, particularly those with CCHS, are able to lead fulfilling lives with appropriate management.

REFERENCES

1. Kc P, Martin RJ. Role of central neurotransmission and chemoreception on airway control. Respir Physiol Neurobiol 2010;173(3):213–22.
2. Nurse CA. Neurotransmitter and neuromodulatory mechanisms at peripheral arterial chemoreceptors. Exp Physiol 2010;95(6):657–67.
3. Forster HV, Smith CA. Contributions of central and peripheral chemoreceptors to the ventilatory response to CO2/H+. J Appl Physiol (1985) 2010; 108(4):989–94.
4. Guyenet PG, Bayliss DA, Stornetta RL, et al. Retrotrapezoid nucleus, respiratory chemosensitivity and breathing automaticity. Respir Physiol Neurobiol 2009;168(1–2):59–68.
5. Gozal D, Kheirandish-Gozal L. Disorders of breathing during sleep. In: Wilmott RW, editor. Kendig and Chernick's disorders of the respiratory tract in children. Philadelphia: Elsevier; 2012. p. 1067–86.
6. Colrain IM, Trinder J, Fraser G, et al. Ventilation during sleep onset. J Appl Physiol 1987;63(5):2067–74.
7. Housley GD. Recent insights into the regulation of breathing. Auton Neurosci 2011;164(1–2):3–5.
8. Richardson HL, Parslow PM, Walker AM, et al. Maturation of the initial ventilatory response to hypoxia in sleeping infants. J Sleep Res 2007;16(1): 117–27.
9. Mellins RB, Balfour HH Jr, Turino GM, et al. Failure of automatic control of ventilation (Ondine's curse). Report of an infant born with this syndrome and review of the literature. Medicine (Baltimore) 1970; 49(6):487–504.
10. Amiel J, Laudier B, Attie-Bitach T, et al. Polyalanine expansion and frameshift mutations of the paired-like homeobox gene PHOX2B in congenital central hypoventilation syndrome. Nat Genet 2003;33(4): 459–61.
11. Weese-Mayer DE, Berry-Kravis EM, Zhou L, et al. Idiopathic congenital central hypoventilation syndrome: analysis of genes pertinent to early autonomic nervous system embryologic development and identification of mutations in PHOX2b. Am J Med Genet A 2003;123(3):267–78.
12. Weese-Mayer DE, Berry-Kravis EM, Ceccherini I, et al. An official ATS clinical policy statement: congenital central hypoventilation syndrome: genetic basis, diagnosis, and management. Am J Respir Crit Care Med 2010;181(6):626–44.
13. Trang H, Dehan M, Beaufils F, et al. The French Congenital Central Hypoventilation Syndrome Registry: general data, phenotype, and genotype. Chest 2005;127(1):72–9.
14. Todd ES, Weinberg SM, Berry-Kravis EM, et al. Facial phenotype in children and young adults with PHOX2B-determined congenital central hypoventilation syndrome: quantitative pattern of dysmorphology. Pediatr Res 2006;59(1):39–45.
15. Paton JY, Swaminathan S, Sargent CW, et al. Ventilatory response to exercise in children with congenital central hypoventilation syndrome. Am Rev Respir Dis 1993;147(5):1185–91.
16. Gozal D, Simakajornboon N. Passive motion of the extremities modifies alveolar ventilation during sleep in patients with congenital central hypoventilation syndrome. Am J Respir Crit Care Med 2000; 162(5):1747–51.
17. Gozal D, Marcus CL, Shoseyov D, et al. Peripheral chemoreceptor function in children with the congenital central hypoventilation syndrome. J Appl Physiol 1993;74(1):379–87.
18. Paton JY, Swaminathan S, Sargent CW, et al. Hypoxic and hypercapnic ventilatory responses in awake children with congenital central hypoventilation syndrome. Am Rev Respir Dis 1989;140(2):368–72.
19. Huang J, Marcus CL, Bandla P, et al. Cortical processing of respiratory occlusion stimuli in children with central hypoventilation syndrome. Am J Respir Crit Care Med 2008;178(7):757–64.
20. Lavorini F, Fontana GA, Pantaleo T, et al. Fog-induced cough with impaired respiratory sensation in congenital central hypoventilation syndrome. Am J Respir Crit Care Med 2007;176(8):825–32.
21. Macey KE, Macey PM, Woo MA, et al. fMRI signal changes in response to forced expiratory loading in congenital central hypoventilation syndrome. J Appl Physiol 2004;97(5):1897–907.
22. Ogren JA, Macey PM, Kumar R, et al. Central autonomic regulation in congenital central hypoventilation syndrome. Neuroscience 2010;167(4): 1249–56.
23. Woo MA, Macey PM, Macey KE, et al. FMRI responses to hyperoxia in congenital central hypoventilation syndrome. Pediatr Res 2005;57(4):510–8.
24. Vanderlaan M, Holbrook CR, Wang M, et al. Epidemiologic survey of 196 patients with congenital central hypoventilation syndrome. Pediatr Pulmonol 2004;37(3):217–29.
25. Fishman LS, Samson JH, Sperling DR. Primary alveolar hypoventilation syndrome (Ondine's Curse). Am J Dis Child 1965;110:155–61.

26. Ize-Ludlow D, Gray JA, Sperling MA, et al. Rapid-onset obesity with hypothalamic dysfunction, hypoventilation, and autonomic dysregulation presenting in childhood. Pediatrics 2007;120(1):e179–88.

27. Katz ES, McGrath S, Marcus CL. Late-onset central hypoventilation with hypothalamic dysfunction: a distinct clinical syndrome. Pediatr Pulmonol 2000; 29(1):62–8.

28. Abaci A, Catli G, Bayram E, et al. A case of rapid-onset obesity with hypothalamic dysfunction, hypoventilation, autonomic dysregulation, and neural crest tumor: ROHHADNET syndrome. Endocr Pract 2013;19(1):e12–6.

29. De Pontual L, Trochet D, Caillat-Zucman S, et al. Delineation of late onset hypoventilation associated with hypothalamic dysfunction syndrome. Pediatr Res 2008;64(6):689–94.

30. Rand CM, Patwari PP, Rodikova EA, et al. Rapid-onset obesity with hypothalamic dysfunction, hypoventilation, and autonomic dysregulation: analysis of hypothalamic and autonomic candidate genes. Pediatr Res 2011;70(4):375–8.

31. Riley CM, Day RL, et al. Central autonomic dysfunction with defective lacrimation; report of five cases. Pediatrics 1949;3(4):468–78.

32. Norcliffe-Kaufmann L, Kaufmann H. Familial dysautonomia (Riley-Day syndrome): when baroreceptor feedback fails. Auton Neurosci 2012; 172(1–2):26–30.

33. Norcliffe-Kaufmann L, Axelrod FB, Kaufmann H. Developmental abnormalities, blood pressure variability and renal disease in Riley Day syndrome. J Hum Hypertens 2013;27(1):51–5.

34. Norcliffe-Kaufmann L, Axelrod F, Kaufmann H. Afferent baroreflex failure in familial dysautonomia. Neurology 2010;75(21):1904–11.

35. Bernardi L, Hilz M, Stemper B, et al. Respiratory and cerebrovascular responses to hypoxia and hypercapnia in familial dysautonomia. Am J Respir Crit Care Med 2003;167(2):141–9.

36. Carroll MS, Kenny AS, Patwari PP, et al. Respiratory and cardiovascular indicators of autonomic nervous system dysregulation in familial dysautonomia. Pediatr Pulmonol 2012;47(7):682–91.

37. Weese-Mayer DE, Kenny AS, Bennett HL, et al. Familial dysautonomia: frequent, prolonged and severe hypoxemia during wakefulness and sleep. Pediatr Pulmonol 2008;43(3):251–60.

38. Axelrod FB, Goldberg JD, Ye XY, et al. Survival in familial dysautonomia: impact of early intervention. J Pediatr 2002;141(4):518–23.

39. Gold-von Simson G, Axelrod FB. Familial dysautonomia: update and recent advances. Curr Probl Pediatr Adolesc Health Care 2006;36(6):218–37.

40. Ngai J, Kreynin I, Kim JT, et al. Anesthesia management of familial dysautonomia. Paediatr Anaesth 2006;16(6):611–20.

41. Adzick NS, Walsh DS. Myelomeningocele: prenatal diagnosis, pathophysiology and management. Semin Pediatr Surg 2003;12(3):168–74.

42. Ward SL, Nickerson BG, van der Hal A, et al. Absent hypoxic and hypercapneic arousal responses in children with myelomeningocele and apnea. Pediatrics 1986;78(1):44–50.

43. Gilbert JN, Jones KL, Rorke LB, et al. Central nervous system anomalies associated with meningomyelocele, hydrocephalus, and the Arnold-Chiari malformation: reappraisal of theories regarding the pathogenesis of posterior neural tube closure defects. Neurosurgery 1986;18(5):559–64.

44. Kirk VG, Morielli A, Gozal D, et al. Treatment of sleep-disordered breathing in children with myelomeningocele. Pediatr Pulmonol 2000;30(6): 445–52.

45. Alsaadi MM, Iqbal SM, Elgamal EA, et al. Sleep-disordered breathing in children with Chiari malformation type II and myelomeningocele. Pediatr Int 2012;54(5):623–6.

46. Sherman MS, Kaplan JM, Effgen S, et al. Pulmonary dysfunction and reduced exercise capacity in patients with myelomeningocele. J Pediatr 1997;131(3):413–8.

47. Hays RM, Jordan RA, McLaughlin JF, et al. Central ventilatory dysfunction in myelodysplasia: an independent determinant of survival. Dev Med Child Neurol 1989;31(3):366–70.

48. Tsara V, Serasli E, Kimiskidis V, et al. Acute respiratory failure and sleep-disordered breathing in Arnold-Chiari malformation. Clin Neurol Neurosurg 2005;107(6):521–4.

49. Murray C, Seton C, Prelog K, et al. Arnold Chiari type 1 malformation presenting with sleep disordered breathing in well children. Arch Dis Child 2006;91(4):342–3.

50. Gosalakkal JA. Sleep-disordered breathing in Chiari malformation type 1. Pediatr Neurol 2008; 39(3):207–8.

51. Yoshimi A, Nomura K, Furune S. Sleep apnea syndrome associated with a type I Chiari malformation. Brain Dev 2002;24(1):49–51.

52. Shiihara T, Shimizu Y, Mitsui T, et al. Isolated sleep apnea due to Chiari type I malformation and syringomyelia. Pediatr Neurol 1995;13(3):266–7.

53. Cassidy SB, Schwartz S, Miller JL, et al. Prader-Willi syndrome. Genet Med 2012;14(1):10–26.

54. Gozal D, Arens R, Omlin KJ, et al. Absent peripheral chemosensitivity in Prader-Willi syndrome. J Appl Physiol 1994;77(5):2231–6.

55. Arens R, Gozal D, Omlin KJ, et al. Hypoxic and hypercapnic ventilatory responses in Prader-Willi syndrome. J Appl Physiol 1994;77(5):2224–30.

56. Livingston FR, Arens R, Bailey SL, et al. Hypercapnic arousal responses in Prader-Willi syndrome. Chest 1995;108(6):1627–31.

57. Arens R, Gozal D, Burrell BC, et al. Arousal and cardiorespiratory responses to hypoxia in Prader-Willi syndrome. Am J Respir Crit Care Med 1996; 153(1):283–7.

58. Festen DA, de Weerd AW, van den Bossche RA, et al. Sleep-related breathing disorders in prepubertal children with Prader-Willi syndrome and effects of growth hormone treatment. J Clin Endocrinol Metab 2006;91(12):4911–5.

59. Al-Saleh S, Al-Naimi A, Hamilton J, et al. Longitudinal evaluation of sleep-disordered breathing in children with Prader-Willi Syndrome during 2 years of growth hormone therapy. J Pediatr 2013;162(2): 263–8.e1.

60. Riedl S, Blumel P, Zwiauer K, et al. Death in two female Prader-Willi syndrome patients during the early phase of growth hormone treatment. Acta Paediatr 2005;94(7):974–7.

61. Grugni G, Livieri C, Corrias A, et al. Death during GH therapy in children with Prader-Willi syndrome: description of two new cases. J Endocrinol Invest 2005;28(6):554–7.

62. Deal CL, Tony M, Hoybye C, et al. Growth Hormone Research Society workshop summary: consensus guidelines for recombinant human growth hormone therapy in Prader-Willi syndrome. J Clin Endocrinol Metab 2013;98(6):E1072–87.

63. Horton WA, Hall JG, Hecht JT. Achondroplasia. Lancet 2007;370(9582):162–72.

64. Wright MJ, Irving MD. Clinical management of achondroplasia. Arch Dis Child 2012;97(2):129–34.

65. Mogayzel PJ Jr, Carroll JL, Loughlin GM, et al. Sleep-disordered breathing in children with achondroplasia. J Pediatr 1998;132(4):667–71.

66. Afsharpaiman S, Saburi A, Waters KA. Respiratory difficulties and breathing disorders in achondroplasia. Paediatr Respir Rev 2013;14(4):250–5.

67. Pauli RM, Scott CI, Wassman ER Jr, et al. Apnea and sudden unexpected death in infants with achondroplasia. J Pediatr 1984;104(3):342–8.

68. Fremion AS, Garg BP, Kalsbeck J. Apnea as the sole manifestation of cord compression in achondroplasia. J Pediatr 1984;104(3):398–401.

69. Stokes DC, Phillips JA, Leonard CO, et al. Respiratory complications of achondroplasia. J Pediatr 1983;102(4):534–41.

70. Colamaria V, Mazza C, Beltramello A, et al. Irreversible respiratory failure in an achondroplastic child: the importance of an early cervicomedullary decompression, and a review of the literature. Brain Dev 1991;13(4):270–9.

71. Finsterer J. Leigh and Leigh-like syndrome in children and adults. Pediatr Neurol 2008;39(4): 223–35.

72. Rosing HS, Hopkins LC, Wallace DC, et al. Maternally inherited mitochondrial myopathy and myoclonic epilepsy. Ann Neurol 1985;17(3):228–37.

73. Johnston K, Newth CJ, Sheu KF, et al. Central hypoventilation syndrome in pyruvate dehydrogenase complex deficiency. Pediatrics 1984;74(6): 1034–40.

74. Barohn RJ, Clanton T, Sahenk Z, et al. Recurrent respiratory insufficiency and depressed ventilatory drive complicating mitochondrial myopathies. Neurology 1990;40(1):103–6.

75. Manni R, Piccolo G, Banfi P, et al. Respiratory patterns during sleep in mitochondrial myopathies with ophthalmoplegia. Eur Neurol 1991;31(1):12–7.

76. Matsuyama M, Nakazawa K, Katou M, et al. Central alveolar hypoventilation syndrome due to surgical resection for bulbar hemangioblastoma. Intern Med 2009;48(11):925–30.

77. Uchino A, Iizuka T, Urano Y, et al. Pseudo-piano playing motions and nocturnal hypoventilation in anti-NMDA receptor encephalitis: response to prompt tumor removal and immunotherapy. Intern Med 2011;50(6):627–30.

78. Hui SH, Wing YK, Poon W, et al. Alveolar hypoventilation syndrome in brainstem glioma with improvement after surgical resection. Chest 2000;118(1): 266–8.

79. Aronow WS, Stemmer EA. Idiopathic alveolar hypoventilation related to head trauma. Chest 1972; 61(2):187–8.

80. Tirupathi S, Webb DW, Phelan E, et al. Central hypoventilation syndrome after Haemophilus influenzae type b meningitis and herpes infection. Pediatr Neurol 2008;39(5):358–60.

81. Goldenberg D, Ari EG, Golz A, et al. Tracheotomy complications: a retrospective study of 1130 cases. Otolaryngol Head Neck Surg 2000;123(4):495–500.

82. Marcus CL, Jansen MT, Poulsen MK, et al. Medical and psychosocial outcome of children with congenital central hypoventilation syndrome. J Pediatr 1991;119(6):888–95.

83. Berry RB, Chediak A, Brown LK, et al. Best clinical practices for the sleep center adjustment of noninvasive positive pressure ventilation (NPPV) in stable chronic alveolar hypoventilation syndromes. J Clin Sleep Med 2010;6(5):491–509.

84. Hartmann H, Jawad MH, Noyes J, et al. Negative extrathoracic pressure ventilation in central hypoventilation syndrome. Arch Dis Child 1994;70(5):418–23.

85. Levy RD, Cosio MG, Gibbons L, et al. Induction of sleep apnoea with negative pressure ventilation in patients with chronic obstructive lung disease. Thorax 1992;47(8):612–5.

86. Weese-Mayer DE, Hunt CE, Brouillette RT, et al. Diaphragm pacing in infants and children. J Pediatr 1992;120(1):1–8.

87. Chen ML, Tablizo MA, Kun S, et al. Diaphragm pacers as a treatment for congenital central hypoventilation syndrome. Expert Rev Med Devices 2005;2(5):577–85.

88. DiMarco AF. Phrenic nerve stimulation in patients with spinal cord injury. Respir Physiol Neurobiol 2009;169(2):200–9.

89. Hyland RH, Hutcheon MA, Perl A, et al. Upper airway occlusion induced by diaphragm pacing for primary alveolar hypoventilation: implications for the pathogenesis of obstructive sleep apnea. Am Rev Respir Dis 1981;124(2):180–5.

90. Antic N, McEvoy RD. Primary alveolar hypoventilation and response to the respiratory stimulant almitrine. Intern Med J 2002;32(12):622–4.

91. Mahmoud M, Bryan Y, Gunter J, et al. Anesthetic implications of undiagnosed late onset central hypoventilation syndrome in a child: from elective tonsillectomy to tracheostomy. Paediatr Anaesth 2007;17(10):1001–5.

92. Ishibashi H, Umezawa K, Hayashi S, et al. Anesthetic management of a child with congenital central hypoventilation syndrome (CCHS, Ondine's curse) for dental treatment. Anesth Prog 2004; 51(3):102–4.

93. Chandrakantan A, Poulton TJ. Anesthetic considerations for rapid-onset obesity, hypoventilation, hypothalamic dysfunction, and autonomic dysfunction (ROHHAD) syndrome in children. Paediatr Anaesth 2013;23(1):28–32.

Central Sleep Apnea in Infants

Salman Raza Khan, MD, Sally L. Davidson Ward, MD*

KEYWORDS

• Central sleep apnea • Infants • Oxygen supplementation • Apnea • Polysomnography

KEY POINTS

- Central apnea (CA) and periodic breathing are common in infants, and are much more common in preterm than term infants.
- Irregular breathing is seen in both active and quiet sleep. It tends to improve with increasing gestational age, and is presumed to be due to maturity of the respiratory control centers and chest-wall mechanics.
- In-laboratory polysomnography is the study of choice for the evaluation of CA in infants. Most therapies directed at treatment of CA are meant to stabilize the breathing pattern and prevent oxygen desaturation.
- Most of these therapies are temporary, and are used for a brief period in preterm and term infants until the breathing matures.

INTRODUCTION

Sleep-disordered breathing encompasses a wide variety of breathing disorders including obstructive sleep apnea, central apnea (CA), and nonobstructive sleep related hypoventilation. Central sleep apnea results from absent respiratory drive from breathing centers in the brainstem during sleep. The criteria that meets the definition of CA differ between children and adults. The American Academy of Sleep Medicine (AASM) defines CA in children as cessation of breathing during sleep without any breathing effort for a duration of 20 seconds or longer, or lasting at least 2 breaths' duration with 3% oxygen desaturation or arousal.[1] In infants, the CA is at least 2 breaths in duration and is associated with a decrease in heart rate to less than 50 beats per minute for at least 5 seconds, or less than 60 beats per minute for 15 seconds. Periodic breathing is a form of CA that has been described as greater than 3 episodes of CA lasting 3 seconds separated by no more than 20 seconds of normal breathing.[1] Apnea following a sigh is not considered pathologic unless it is associated with arousal or desaturation. Isolated central sleep apnea (**Fig. 1**A), CA following sigh breathing (see **Fig. 1**B), CA following body movements, and periodic breathing patterns (see **Fig. 1**C) can be seen in healthy infants and children.[2] It is common to see CA in healthy infants, but on rare occasions it can be a harbinger of ominous pathologic consequences, such as congenital central hypoventilation syndrome or Arnold-Chiari malformation.[3] The severity of CA can be characterized using the apnea-hypopnea index (AHI), the total number of events overnight divided by hours of sleep. There is no clear description in the literature of pathologic central AHI, but studies have considered a central AHI from greater than 0.9 to AHI greater than 5 as abnormal.[4–6] The adverse consequences of moderate and severe CA are well known, but those of CA of milder degree is still debated.[7] The mild CA seen in otherwise healthy infants tends to improve with age, and older children can have rare CAs.[5,8] The improvement in apnea frequency can be considered as maturation of respiratory control and chest-wall mechanics.

Division of Pediatric Pulmonology, Children's Hospital Los Angeles, 4650 Sunset Boulevard, Los Angeles, CA 90027, USA
* Corresponding author. 4650 Sunset Boulevard, Mail Stop #83, Los Angeles, CA 90027.
E-mail address: Sward@chla.usc.edu

Sleep Med Clin 9 (2014) 119–129
http://dx.doi.org/10.1016/j.jsmc.2013.10.009
1556-407X/14/$ – see front matter © 2014 Elsevier Inc. All rights reserved

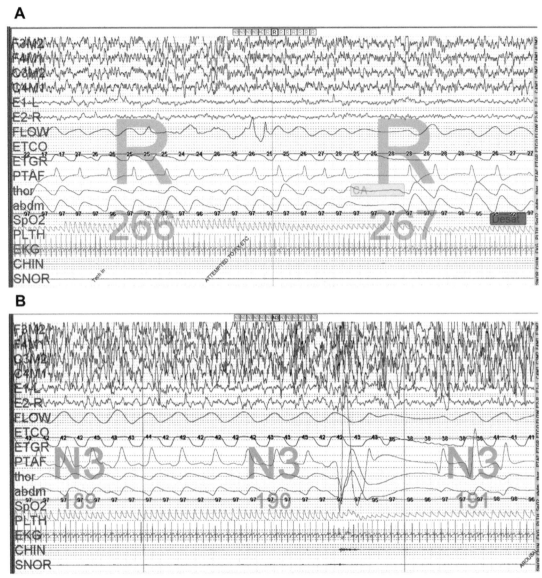

Fig. 1. (*A–C*) Sixty-second-long epoch of the polysomnography of a 21-month-old child born at full term, referred for evaluation of sleep apnea because of a family history of sudden infant death syndrome. (*A*) Central sleep apnea without arousal. (*B*) Central sleep apnea after arousal during stage 3 non–rapid eye movement sleep. (*C*) Periodic breathing during rapid eye movement sleep. abdm, abdominal plethysmography; C3, C4, central electroencephalogram leads; CHIN, chin electromyogram; E1, left eye electromyogram; E2, right eye electromyogram; EKG, electrocardiogram; ETCO, end-tidal carbon dioxide tracing; ETGR, End tidal graphical representation; F3, F4, frontal electroencephalogram leads; FLOW, tracing of oral thermistor; PLTH, Plethysmography; PTAF, for measurement of nasal air flow; SNOR, snore micrograph; SpO2, continuous pulse oximetry; thor, thoracic plethysmography.

APNEA IN HEALTHY NORMAL INFANTS

Brief CA in full-term infants is very common, especially in the early months of life. The duration and frequency of CA improves with age.[9,10] Several studies have focused on defining the prevalence of CA in healthy infants. Each study has used different criteria to define CA, different monitoring techniques, and different testing environments such as home versus in-laboratory polysomnography, which makes it difficult to make comparisons between the studies. As already noted, standardization of the definition of CA has been achieved, which will make interstudy comparisons in the future much easier and more fruitful. Home monitoring provides an opportunity to collect data in infants during sleep for a long

C

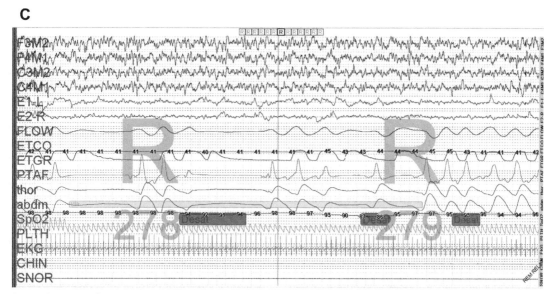

Fig. 1. (*continued*)

period in familiar surroundings. The limitations of home monitoring include inability to assess the exact duration of apnea caused by lack of airflow, and reliance on breathing pattern and heart rate to differentiate between sleep and wakefulness. The Collaborative Home Infant Monitoring Evaluation (CHIME) study is perhaps the most comprehensive study allowing comparison of breathing patterns during sleep in healthy term infants, siblings of infants with a family history of sudden infant death syndrome (SIDS), healthy preterm infants, and infants with apparent life-threatening events (ALTE) in both term and preterm subjects.[11] The study was conducted in almost 1100 infants over 6 months' duration in their home environment. The investigators concluded that conventional events, described as apnea of 20 seconds' duration not associated with bradycardia, are not uncommon in otherwise healthy term infants. The study also reported that extreme events, described as apneas longer than 30 seconds associated with bradycardia, are more common in premature infants and tend to reduce in frequency after 43 weeks gestational age (GA). A strength of the study is the ability to potentially differentiate between central, obstructive, and mixed apneas.[12] In another smaller study, breathing was monitored in the home environment in healthy term infants for a shorter period.[9] Electrocardiography (ECG) and abdominal-wall movement was used to define apnea in 110 subjects, and subjects were monitored at 2, 6, 12, and 24 weeks of age. It was concluded that CAs of longer than 20 seconds are common

in first 2 weeks of life, and rare afterward. Periodic breathing was seen in all age groups studied, and improved with age.

In another study of 46 full-term healthy infants, the investigators used pneumograms, overnight recording of the respiratory pattern by impedance and heart-rate monitoring, to define the incidence of CA in the nursery and home settings.[13] The recordings were made at birth, 1 month, and 3 months of age. A modified definition of CA, with duration of 5 seconds, was used. There was no mention of desaturation association with apnea, nor was there any characterization of sleep and wakefulness. The investigators relied on parents' descriptions of sleep and wakefulness, and reported that apnea of longer than 15 seconds at birth and 4 weeks of age is rare. Moreover, there was significant intersubject and intrasubject variability in terms of apnea frequency, pattern of apnea, and change in pattern of apnea over the first 4 weeks of life.

In-laboratory monitoring for sleep-disordered breathing is also associated with limitations and advantages. The data collected during this monitoring is for a shorter duration but has better ability to characterize events such as non–rapid eye movement (NREM) sleep, rapid eye movement (REM) sleep, and wakefulness. In a smaller study of 9 full-term infants, the investigators studied subjects in a laboratory setting at monthly intervals until 6 months of age,[10] using slightly different criteria to define apnea and periodic breathing. CA was defined as of at least 6 seconds' duration, while periodic breathing was at least 2 CAs alternating with regular breathing of at least 3 seconds in a 20-second period. The investigators reported that CA is common until 3 months of age and that it is rare to see CA of 15 seconds' duration afterward. The frequency of apnea decreases after 3 months. Most apneas were in active sleep (ie, REM sleep). It was further reported that periodic breathing remained stable across the ages and was mostly seen in active sleep.

In an attempt to describe normative data of breathing patterns during sleep in older children, Uliel and colleagues[5] studied 70 subjects between the ages of 1 and 15 years who underwent a single-night sleep study in the laboratory. CA was defined as of at least 10 seconds' duration or any duration associated with desaturation of greater than 4% compared with baseline. The investigators confirmed that CA is rare in children, and stated that CA with desaturation is even rarer. The study was conducted with a modern computer-based recording system and was manually scored by visual inspection.

On review of the literature, it can be suggested that CA is common in early infancy and improves with age. It is also rare to see CA not following a sigh breath in older healthy children beyond infancy. One should keep in mind that these studies used different monitoring techniques, variable duration of monitoring periods, different testing environments, and variability in describing CA in the population tested. These differences limit the ability to compare studies.

APNEA OF PREMATURITY

Central apnea and periodic breathing in premature infants is a rule rather than an exception. With the technological advancement in the neonatal intensive care unit (NICU) and the availability of newer and improved medications, extremely premature infants are surviving. The etiology of premature birth is multifactorial, but results in the birth of an infant who is not fully equipped to transition to an independent life. The premature birth results in significant comorbidity and mortality later in life that compounds the difficulty in transition to postnatal life. In premature infants, the breathing pattern is not fully developed at the time of birth.[14] This situation may be complicated with the development of bronchopulmonary dysplasia with limited respiratory reserves, and/or cerebral palsy with associated poor neuromuscular control of upper airway.[15] Thus, prematurity predisposes to both central and obstructive sleep apnea. Most studies performed in premature infants to assess the maturation of breathing are retrospective in nature.

In a retrospective study, Eichenwald and colleagues[16] reviewed the medical records of 457 subjects born between 24 and 28 weeks GA to assess the natural history of recurrent apnea and bradycardia in premature infants. The nursing documentation of apnea alarms and the infants' condition were reviewed. The monitor alarm was set for apnea duration of 20 seconds, and bradycardia for a heart rate less than 100 beats/min in infants younger than 35 weeks GA and less than 80 beats/min thereafter. The investigators found that apnea and bradycardia were reported in all infants. The time to resolution of apnea was longer for infants born at lower GA. Infants born between 24 and 27 weeks GA had recurrent apnea and bradycardia at 36 and 38 weeks but not beyond 40 weeks GA, compared with those born at 28 weeks GA. Later resolution of recurrent apnea and bradycardia was strongly correlated with higher incidence of chronic lung disease, but not with severity of head ultrasonographic abnormalities. The study is limited because of its inability to characterize types of apnea based on the NICU monitor and to differentiate sleep and wakefulness, and its retrospective nature.

In yet another retrospective study, investigators reviewed the charts of 865 infants born between 24 and 32 weeks GA to assess the maturity of different body functions including breathing patterns.[17] Nurse-documented monitor events were used to characterize apnea and bradycardia. The monitor alarm was set for an apnea duration of 20 seconds and bradycardia of less than 80 beats/min. The investigators reported that at 31 weeks GA 25% of patients were free of apnea and bradycardia, and by 36 weeks GA all were without apnea or bradycardia. Furthermore, infants born at less than 26 weeks GA demonstrated a delay in becoming apnea free by a mean of 2.3 weeks when compared with infants born at 31 and 32 weeks GA. Bronchopulmonary dysplasia and necrotizing enterocolitis were associated with a delay in becoming apnea and bradycardia free.

Periodic breathing is also common in premature infants (**Fig. 2**). In an attempt to describe the prevalence of periodic breathing in relatively mature preterm infants (30–35 weeks GA) in comparison with full-term infants, Glotzbach and colleagues[18] recorded pneumograms in 66 preterm infants before discharge. The investigators reported a higher mean percentage value of periodic breathing per quiet sleep and number of episodes of periodic breathing per 100 minutes of quiet sleep, and the longest episode of periodic breathing was higher in preterm infants than in full-term controls. Moreover, percentage and episodes of

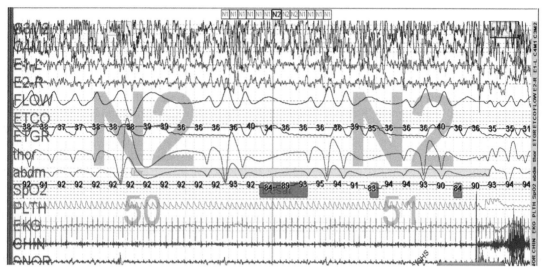

Fig. 2. Sixty-second-long epoch of the polysomnography in a 6-month-old child with periodic breathing born at 26 weeks gestational age. abdm, abdominal plethysmography; C3, C4, central electroencephalogram leads; CHIN, chin electromyogram; E1, left eye electromyogram; E2, right eye electromyogram; EKG, electrocardiogram; ETCO, end-tidal carbon dioxide tracing; ETGR, End tidal graphical representation; FLOW, tracing of oral thermistor; PLTH, Plethysmography; SNOR, snore micrograph; SpO2, continuous pulse oximetry; thor, thoracic plethysmography.

periodic breathing during sleep decreased as infants reached 39 to 41 weeks postgestational age. The study suggests that periodic breathing is common in premature infants and decreases as infants approach term GA. Periodic breathing is also seen in full-term infants.

APPARENT LIFE-THREATENING EVENT

ALTE has been described as an episode that is frightening to the observer and characterized by some combination of apnea, color change, marked change in muscle tone, choking, and/or gagging. The pathophysiology of ALTE is multifactorial; occasionally it is a single event, and no significant pathologic features may be discovered despite extensive investigation.[19] In the past, it was proposed that some infants who die of SIDS had recurrent ALTE, but most patients with ALTE do not die.[20–24] The true prevalence of ALTE is difficult to assess because of the wide range of definitions used to describe ALTE, geographic variations in care, and different patient populations studied.[25,26] It is further complicated because the definition involves the caregiver response to the particular event, which is variable; some parents perhaps ignore the event completely, whereas others may misperceive normal physiologic body function as abnormal.

There are various of causes for ALTE, and it is difficult to focus on a single system function.[27]

Several retrospective studies have focused on different organ systems involved in infants who survived ALTE and underwent extensive workup. Most of these studies failed to show any significant abnormalities discovered during the initial workup, but some studies have suggested that patients with ALTE should have close follow-up, as the chances of missing any neurologic disease may be high on initial workup.[28,29–31] Child abuse has been reported as a cause of ALTE Munchausen by proxy, and these children are at higher risk of death subsequently.[32,33] A few studies highlight that the autonomic nervous system may be abnormal in infants who have suffered ALTE.[34–36]

Apnea may not necessarily be part of the presentation in infants who present with ALTE. The AASM recommends performing polysomnography in infants with clinical suspicion of sleep-disordered breathing.[37] The studies that have assessed sleep-disordered breathing as an etiologic factor in ALTE have used various techniques and different populations of subjects, which make it difficult to draw conclusions. The early studies implicated CA as a major cause of SIDS but only in a very limited number of patients studied.[13] In a study of 340 infants who experienced an ALTE a pneumogram was performed, with subsequent home monitoring in infants with abnormal pneumograms. Rahilly[23] reported that 8% of subjects had abnormal findings, and most these infants had CA on home monitoring.

In a study of infants who were admitted with ALTE, extreme respiratory events, described as CA of 30 seconds' duration or bradycardia of longer than 20 seconds, are more likely to be associated with upper respiratory infection, premature birth, and GA of less than 43 weeks.[38] To delineate the relationship between gastroesophageal reflux (GER) and apnea, Khan and colleagues[39] studied both central and obstructive apnea in 50 infants with ALTE and 50 control subjects. It was concluded that there is no temporal association between GER in the middle esophagus and apnea/bradycardia in both populations. Periodic breathing has also been shown in excessive amounts in patients with ALTE.[40] It is unclear whether CA or periodic breathing is associated with or is a cause of ALTE in infants, and the relationship between ALTE and SIDS is less than tenuous at best.[41]

In a recent prospective study of 300 infants who presented with ALTE and underwent pneumography, Mittal and colleagues[42] showed that the presence of abnormal pneumographic findings does not predict recurrent ALTE.

PATHOPHYSIOLOGY OF CENTRAL APNEA IN INFANTS

The exact timing of the start of breathing movements in the human fetus is unclear, but most of the data derived from animal models show that it starts fairly early in fetal life. It is suggested that fetal breathing movement in most mammals starts in the second trimester.[43] The role of breathing is not gas exchange in fetal life, this being achieved via the circulatory system and placenta. The fetal breathing movement is noncontinuous, rhythmic, and nonsynchronized.[44] During periods of high-voltage, low-frequency activity, electrocorticography of the fetus is apneic (similarly to REM sleep).[45] Perhaps an important aspect of breathing rhythm in the fetus is that it is vital for lung development during fetal life.[46] The control of breathing in fetal life is complex, and involves several inhibitory and excitatory stimuli. Some of the important modulators of breathing include central rhythm generators, central and peripheral chemoreceptors, sleep and wake states, and various neurotransmitters.[47,48]

Based on the animal model of respiratory control, there are 2 distinct groups of respiratory centers that function in harmony. The first, the parafacial nucleus, is located at the ventral surface of the hindbrain while the second, the pre-Bötzinger complex, is on the dorsal aspect. Both groups of neurons develop independently from each other in the hindbrain.[49] The parafacial nucleus predominantly controls expiration and functions by phasic inhibition of tonic background inspiratory activity via glutamatergic neurons.[50] The pre-Bötzinger complex predominately works as the inspiratory control. The development of these respiratory centers and the interaction between them is beyond the scope of this review.

Fetal breathing is stimulated with elevated carbon dioxide during low-voltage high-frequency electrocorticography, suggestive of awake state, and during both high-voltage and low-voltage electrocorticography with exposure to cold and carbon dioxide.[51,52] Responses to hypoxia and hypercapnia in fetal life suggest that carotid chemoreceptors are already active in fetal life.[53] A powerful inhibitory effect of the upper lateral pons may be responsible for the episodic nature of fetal breathing.[54] The other inhibitory stimuli for breathing in fetal life include adenosine and the placenta.[55,56] Removal of placenta after birth may be a stimulus for continuous breathing.[57] Fetal breathing is also under behavioral control. It is stimulated during high-frequency, low-voltage electrocorticographic activity, which is characteristic of awake and REM sleep, and is inhibited during low-frequency, high-voltage electrocorticographic activity, with apnea being present.[45]

Transition from fetal to neonatal life is probably the most complex transition in human life.[58] In a preterm infant, the transition is difficult because of the immaturity of organ systems, such as an immature breathing pattern and limited lung development that can adapt to an independent life. The intermittent breathing pattern noted in fetal life persists in premature infants and even extends into the age at which they reach term gestation.[59] The irregular breathing pattern in preterm and term infants is also exacerbated by immature lung mechanics at the time of birth. Infants have low functional residual capacity, which results in hypoxemia even with brief CA and periodic breathing.

In premature infants the breathing is irregular, and is characterized by apnea and periodic breathing. Irregular breathing is most commonly seen in active sleep/REM sleep, with breathing becoming more regular during quiet or NREM sleep.[60] The breathing irregularities increase from 30 to 36 weeks GA and then decrease. In full-term infants, breathing irregularities persist during 60% to 70% of the sleep time and decrease by 3 months of age.[61] Warm temperature induces apnea in term infants, and loss of body heat stimulates breathing.[62]

Periodic breathing in premature infants is related to the carbon dioxide level and its relationship to the apnea threshold. Reduction in serum carbon dioxide below a certain point causes apnea during sleep, and this level is termed the apneic threshold. In premature infants, the apnea threshold is much closer to the eucapnia level in comparison with adults.[63] The apnea threshold is therefore frequently reached with common maneuvers such as an augmented breath, resulting in recurrent apnea that is seen in periodic breathing. Another concept in understanding periodic breathing may be related to loop gain, an engineering term. Loop gain is described as a negative feedback system in which a disturbance (u) increases alveolar ventilation from a steady state. This increase in ventilation in turn reduces carbon dioxide, which evokes a negative corrective action (e) to suppress the disturbance. The ratio of e/u will define the loop gain of the system. In the high loop-gain system, the response is greater or equal to the disturbance, which results in an unstable system. For example, a sigh produces a sudden reduction of carbon dioxide levels, which evokes an exaggerated response from the central respiratory center and induces apnea, which in turn results in elevated levels of carbon dioxide. This process causes resumption of breathing but in an exaggerated fashion, leading to washout of carbon dioxide, bringing it below the apneic threshold; the cycle will thus repeat itself, resulting in the characteristic breathing pattern seen in periodic breathing.

DIAGNOSIS

Premature infants often have a prolonged stay in the NICU after birth for respiratory support and nutritional needs. CA and periodic breathing are seen after invasive ventilation has been discontinued. The apnea events may be noticed by the health care staff during routine care and mostly during sleep. Alternatively, the alarm at the bedside will show apnea, bradycardia, and/or desaturation.[64] The accuracy of diagnosis of CA based on nursing documentation is debatable.[65] Patients may have skin-color change and may lose muscle tone. Typically, stimulation will restore breathing in most of the infants. Sometimes the apnea and periodic breathing may be significant enough to require invasive and noninvasive ventilation or oxygen supplementation. After discharge, the premature infants may present with ALTE. Infants with chronic lung disease attributable to prematurity are more likely to have desaturations and apnea events, probably related to the limited respiratory reserves in such infants.[66] The CA is most likely noticed during sleep and rarely during wakefulness. Young infants take frequent naps during the day, so

CA is more likely to be noticed by parents during the day than at night.

Polysomnography is considered a test of choice to diagnose sleep-disordered breathing in infants and children. The study requires in-laboratory testing, which is well tolerated by patients and family members.[67] A recent study has shown that a shorter 4-hour evening study is comparable with an overnight sleep study in the diagnosis of sleep-disordered breathing in children younger than 2 years.[68] A nap study, even shorter than a 4-hour study, is not considered to be equivalent to a full-night study and may miss sleep-disordered breathing.[69] The advantage of in-laboratory polysomnography includes accurate diagnosis of the nature of sleep-disordered breathing, assessment of additional sleep-related physiologic parameters such as sleep-related hypoventilation, and ability to intervene during the study as indicated. The disadvantages include the short period of data collection, expensive testing, and long waiting time for the study because of the shortage of child-friendly sleep laboratories.

Home monitoring has been used in several research studies to document sleep-disordered breathing in infants,[11] but has not been widely accepted as a tool for clinical use. There are various portable testing modalities available for the assessment of sleep-disordered breathing in infants, including home pulse oximetry, pulse transit time, and multichannel unattended sleep studies.[70,71] Portable monitoring provides the advantage to collect data in a patient's familiar surroundings and for an extended period of time. It is also inexpensive and readily available. The disadvantages include difficulty in accurate differentiation of sleep and wake stages, and multiple artifacts during the data collection. Despite these disadvantages, home monitoring for sleep apnea is a valuable tool in certain circumstances.

MANAGEMENT OF CENTRAL APNEA IN INFANTS

Management of CA in infants is aimed at normalization of breathing and stabilization of fluctuation in oxygen saturation. Various therapies are available for the treatment of apnea in infants, but all serve as temporary therapies while awaiting maturity of the breathing apparatus of premature and full-term infants.

Supplemental oxygen is probably the most widely prescribed therapy for CA and periodic breathing in both premature and full-term infants. In a small study of 15 preterm infants, supplemental oxygen improved apnea and periodic breathing.[72] Oxygen therapy prevents desaturation and improves breathing stability in infants. Despite widespread use of supplemental oxygen, there is no clear guideline for its use in the treatment of CA in infants.

Another widely accepted therapy for CA and periodic breathing in preterm and term infants is theophylline or caffeine. In premature infants, the use of caffeine to stimulate breathing is targeted toward adenosine-induced breathing suppression that is normally seen in fetal life.[55] A meta-analysis of 6 clinical trials looking at the efficacy of methylxanthine in the treatment of apnea of prematurity reported a reduction in apnea severity and utilization of intermittent positive pressure therapy in the first 2 to 7 days.[73] In a randomized placebo-controlled trial of 2000 infants born at preterm and with apnea of prematurity, caffeine reduced the need for positive pressure ventilation and reduced the use of supplemental oxygen.[74] The same investigators studied the long-term effect of caffeine used for the treatment of apnea of prematurity, and showed that it reduces the incidence of cerebral palsy and cognitive delay.[75] Caffeine therapy is generally not indicated beyond 33 weeks GA.[76]

Other available nonconventional therapies for the treatment of CA have been researched in preterm infants. A small study of 24 premature infants born at 27 weeks GA with apnea of prematurity compared supine versus prone positioning, and concluded that more CA and less arousal was noted during prone sleeping position, whereas infants had more awakening and arousals per hour in a supine sleeping position.[77] However, a prone sleeping position is a risk factor for SIDS, so this therapy cannot be recommended. In a short, randomized controlled trial of 87 preterm infants born between 27 and 32 weeks GA, Alvaro and colleagues[78] compared theophylline and 1% inhaled carbon dioxide for the treatment of apnea of prematurity. The investigators concluded that theophylline, which was better in reducing the severity of apnea, and carbon dioxide should not be considered as a therapy at this time. In another prospective, randomized controlled study of 27 preterm infants of similar GA, the short-term inhalation of 0.8% carbon dioxide had efficacy similar to that of theophylline in reducing the apnea.[79] Both of these trials were based on the fact that inhaled carbon dioxide will increase the carbon dioxide levels and prevent the apnea threshold being reaching in preterm infants, thus stabilizing breathing.

Positive pressure ventilation has been widely used in the treatment of CA and periodic breathing in preterm and term infants. Continuous positive airway pressure (CPAP) is one such modality. The underlying mechanism of improvement of CA was recently studied by Edwards and colleagues[80] in a lamb model of periodic breathing. CPAP reduced CA and mixed apnea in a dose-dependent manner, most likely by reducing the loop gain via an increase in the lung volume.

Other therapies that have been studied in preterm infants for treatment of CA and periodic breathing, but not yet available for clinical use, include stochastic mechanosensory stimulation (vibrotactile stimulation to stimulate breathing). In a small study of 10 relatively mature preterm infants (33 weeks), a low level of exogenous stochastic stimulation stabilized breathing during sleep and helped to reduce the incidence of apnea and periodic breathing.[81] Acetazolamide, a carbonic anhydrase inhibitor, has been used in treatment of CA and periodic breathing. In a small study of 12 infants with recurrent hypoxemia, acetazolamide reduced the CA index and improved oxygen saturation.[82] Treatment of anemia of prematurity with blood transfusion has also been shown to reduce central apnea in preterm infants.[83]

SUMMARY

CA and periodic breathing are common in infants, and are much more common in preterm than in term infants. The irregular breathing is seen in both active and quiet sleep. Irregular breathing tends to improve with increasing GA, and is presumed to be due to maturity of the respiratory control centers and chest-wall mechanics. In-laboratory polysomnography is the study of choice for the evaluation of CA in infants. Most therapies directed at the treatment of CA are aimed at stabilizing the breathing pattern and preventing oxygen desaturation. Most of these therapies are temporary, and are used for a brief period in preterm and term infants until the breathing matures.

REFERENCES

1. Berry RB, Budhiraja R, Gottlieb DJ, et al. Rules for scoring respiratory events in sleep: update of the 2007 AASM Manual for the Scoring of Sleep and Associated Events. Deliberations of the Sleep Apnea Definitions Task Force of the American Academy of Sleep Medicine. J Clin Sleep Med 15;8(5):597–619.
2. Fukumizu M, Kohyama J. Central respiratory pauses, sighs, and gross body movements during sleep in children. Physiol Behav 2004;82(4):721–6.
3. Weese-Mayer DE, Berry-Kravis EM, Ceccherini I, et al. An official ATS clinical policy statement: congenital central hypoventilation syndrome: genetic

basis, diagnosis, and management. Am J Respir Crit Care Med 2010;181(6):626–44.

4. Ng DK, Chan CH. A review of normal values of infant sleep polysomnography. Pediatr Neonatol 2013;54(2):82–7.

5. Uliel S, Tauman R, Greenfeld M, et al. Normal polysomnographic respiratory values in children and adolescents. Chest 2004;125(3):872–8.

6. Kritzinger FE, Al-Saleh S, Narang I. Descriptive analysis of central sleep apnea in childhood at a single center. Pediatr Pulmonol 2011;46(10):1023–30.

7. O'Driscoll DM, Foster AM, Ng ML, et al. Central apnoeas have significant effects on blood pressure and heart rate in children. J Sleep Res 2009;18(4):415–21.

8. Marcus CL, Omlin KJ, Basinki DJ, et al. Normal polysomnographic values for children and adolescents. Am Rev Respir Dis 1992;146(5 Pt 1):1235–9.

9. Richards JM, Alexander JR, Shinebourne EA, et al. Sequential 22-hour profiles of breathing patterns and heart rate in 110 full-term infants during their first 6 months of life. Pediatrics 1984;74(5):763–77.

10. Hoppenbrouwers T, Hodgman JE, Harper RM, et al. Polygraphic studies of normal infants during the first six months of life: III. Incidence of apnea and periodic breathing. Pediatrics 1977;60(4):418–25.

11. Ramanathan R, Corwin MJ, Hunt CE, et al. Cardiorespiratory events recorded on home monitors: comparison of healthy infants with those at increased risk for SIDS. JAMA 2001;285(17):2199–207.

12. Weese-Mayer DE, Corwin MJ, Peucker MR, et al. Comparison of apnea identified by respiratory inductance plethysmography with that detected by end-tidal CO_2 or thermistor. The CHIME Study Group. Am J Respir Crit Care Med 2000;162(2 Pt 1):471–80.

13. Steinschneider A. Prolonged apnea and the sudden infant death syndrome: clinical and laboratory observations. Pediatrics 1972;50(4):646–54.

14. Robertson CM, Watt MJ, Dinu IA. Outcomes for the extremely premature infant: what is new? And where are we going? Pediatr Neurol 2009;40(3):189–96.

15. Baraldi E, Filippone M. Chronic lung disease after premature birth. N Engl J Med 2007;357(19):1946–55.

16. Eichenwald EC, Aina A, Stark AR. Apnea frequently persists beyond term gestation in infants delivered at 24 to 28 weeks. Pediatrics 1997;100(3 Pt 1):354–9.

17. Bakewell-Sachs S, Medoff-Cooper B, Escobar GJ, et al. Infant functional status: the timing of physiologic maturation of premature infants. Pediatrics 2009;123(5):e878–86.

18. Glotzbach SF, Baldwin RB, Lederer NE, et al. Periodic breathing in preterm infants: incidence and characteristics. Pediatrics 1989;84(5):785–92.

19. Samuels MP, Poets CF, Noyes JP, et al. Diagnosis and management after life threatening events in infants and young children who received cardiopulmonary resuscitation. BMJ 1993;306(6876):489–92.

20. Infantile Apnea and Home Monitoring. NIH Consens Statement Online 1986 Sep 29-Oct 1;6(6):1-10. Available at: http://consensus.nih.gov/1986/1986InfantApneaMonitoring058html.htm.

21. Rahilly PM. Review of 'near-miss' sudden infant death syndrome and results of simplified pneumographic studies. Aust Paediatr J 1986;22(Suppl 1):53–4.

22. Esani N, Hodgman JE, Ehsani N, et al. Apparent life-threatening events and sudden infant death syndrome: comparison of risk factors. J Pediatr 2008;152(3):365–70.

23. Rahilly PM. The pneumographic and medical investigation of infants suffering apparent life threatening episodes. J Paediatr Child Health 1991;27(6):349–53.

24. Kant S, Fisher JD, Nelson DG, et al. Mortality after discharge in clinically stable infants admitted with a first-time apparent life-threatening event. Am J Emerg Med 2013;31(4):730–3.

25. Semmekrot BA, van Sleuwen BE, Engelberts AC, et al. Surveillance study of apparent life-threatening events (ALTE) in the Netherlands. Eur J Pediatr 2010;169(2):229–36.

26. Ponsonby AL, Dwyer T, Couper D. Factors related to infant apnoea and cyanosis: a population-based study. J Paediatr Child Health 1997;33(4):317–23.

27. McGovern MC, Smith MB. Causes of apparent life threatening events in infants: a systematic review. Arch Dis Child 2004;89(11):1043–8.

28. Claudius I, Keens T. Do all infants with apparent life-threatening events need to be admitted? Pediatrics 2007;119(4):679–83.

29. Mittal MK, Shofer FS, Baren JM. Serious bacterial infections in infants who have experienced an apparent life-threatening event. Ann Emerg Med 2009;54(4):523–7.

30. Hoki R, Bonkowsky JL, Minich LL, et al. Cardiac testing and outcomes in infants after an apparent life-threatening event. Arch Dis Child 2012;97(12):1034–8.

31. Bonkowsky JL, Guenther E, Filloux FM, et al. Death, child abuse, and adverse neurological outcome of infants after an apparent life-threatening event. Pediatrics 2008;122(1):125–31.

32. Guenther E, Powers A, Srivastava R, et al. Abusive head trauma in children presenting with an apparent life-threatening event. J Pediatr 2010;157(5):821–5.

33. Parker K, Pitetti R. Mortality and child abuse in children presenting with apparent life-threatening events. Pediatr Emerg Care 2011;27(7):591–5.

34. Harrington C, Kirjavainen T, Teng A, et al. Altered autonomic function and reduced arousability in apparent life-threatening event infants with obstructive sleep apnea. Am J Respir Crit Care Med 2002;165(8):1048–54.

35. Tirosh E, Ariov-Antebi N, Cohen A. Autonomic function, gastroesophageal reflux in apparent life threatening event. Clin Auton Res 2010;20(3):161–6.

36. Edner A, Ericson M, Milerad J, et al. Abnormal heart rate response to hypercapnia in boys with an apparent life-threatening event. Acta Paediatr 2002;91(12):1318–23.

37. Aurora RN, Zak RS, Karippot A, et al. Practice parameters for the respiratory indications for polysomnography in children. Sleep 2011;34(3):379–88.

38. Al-Kindy HA, Gelinas JF, Hatzakis G, et al. Risk factors for extreme events in infants hospitalized for apparent life-threatening events. J Pediatr 2009;154(3):332–7, 337.e1–2.

39. Kahn A, Rebuffat E, Sottiaux M, et al. Lack of temporal relation between acid reflux in the proximal oesophagus and cardiorespiratory events in sleeping infants. Eur J Pediatr 1992;151(3):208–12.

40. Kelly DH, Shannon DC. Periodic breathing in infants with near-miss sudden infant death syndrome. Pediatrics 1979;63(3):355–60.

41. Fleming P, Tsogt B, Blair PS. Modifiable risk factors, sleep environment, developmental physiology and common polymorphisms: understanding and preventing sudden infant deaths. Early Hum Dev 2006;82(12):761–6.

42. Mittal MK, Donda K, Baren JM. Role of pneumography and esophageal pH monitoring in the evaluation of infants with apparent life-threatening event: a prospective observational study. Clin Pediatr (Phila) 2013;52(4):338–43.

43. Jansen AH, Chernick V. Development of respiratory control. Physiol Rev 1983;63(2):437–83.

44. Johnston BM, Gunn TR, Gluckman PD. Surface cooling rapidly induces coordinated activity in the upper and lower airway muscles of the fetal lamb in utero. Pediatr Res 1988;23(3):257–61.

45. Dawes GS, Fox HE, Leduc BM, et al. Respiratory movements and rapid eye movement sleep in the foetal lamb. J Physiol 1972;220(1):119–43.

46. Wallen-Mackenzie A, Gezelius H, Thoby-Brisson M, et al. Vesicular glutamate transporter 2 is required for central respiratory rhythm generation but not for locomotor central pattern generation. J Neurosci 2006;26(47):12294–307.

47. Corcoran AE, Hodges MR, Wu Y, et al. Medullary serotonin neurons and central CO_2 chemoreception. Respir Physiol Neurobiol 2009;168(1–2):49–58.

48. Wong-Riley MT, Liu Q. Neurochemical development of brain stem nuclei involved in the control of respiration. Respir Physiol Neurobiol 2005;149(1–3):83–98.

49. Bouvier J, Thoby-Brisson M, Renier N, et al. Hindbrain interneurons and axon guidance signaling critical for breathing. Nat Neurosci 2010;13(9):1066–74.

50. Janczewski WA, Feldman JL. Distinct rhythm generators for inspiration and expiration in the juvenile rat. J Physiol 2006;570(Pt 2):407–20.

51. Rigatto H, Lee D, Davi M, et al. Effect of increased arterial CO2 on fetal breathing and behavior in sheep. J Appl Physiol 1988;64(3):982–7.

52. Kuipers IM, Maertzdorf WJ, De Jong DS, et al. The effect of hypercapnia and hypercapnia associated with central cooling on breathing in unanesthetized fetal lambs. Pediatr Res 1997;41(1):90–5.

53. Blanco CE, Dawes GS, Hanson MA, et al. The response to hypoxia of arterial chemoreceptors in fetal sheep and new-born lambs. J Physiol 1984;351:25–37.

54. Gluckman PD, Johnston BM. Lesions in the upper lateral pons abolish the hypoxic depression of breathing in unanaesthetized fetal lambs in utero. J Physiol 1987;382:373–83.

55. Adamson SL, Kuipers IM, Olson DM. Umbilical cord occlusion stimulates breathing independent of blood gases and pH. J Appl Physiol 1991;70(4):1796–809.

56. Koos BJ, Maeda T, Jan C. Adenosine A(1) and A(2A) receptors modulate sleep state and breathing in fetal sheep. J Appl Physiol 2001;91(1):343–50.

57. Alvaro R, de Almeida V, al-Alaiyan S, et al. A placental extract inhibits breathing induced by umbilical cord occlusion in fetal sheep. J Dev Physiol 1993;19(1):23–8.

58. Hillman NH, Kallapur SG, Jobe AH. Physiology of transition from intrauterine to extrauterine life. Clin Perinatol 2012;39(4):769–83.

59. Rigatto H. Regulation of fetal breathing. Reprod Fertil Dev 1996;8(1):23–33.

60. Don GW, Waters KA. Influence of sleep state on frequency of swallowing, apnea, and arousal in human infants. J Appl Physiol 2003;94(6):2456–64.

61. Parmelee AH, Stern E, Harris MA. Maturation of respiration in prematures and young infants. Neuropadiatrie 1972;3(3):294–304.

62. Tourneux P, Cardot V, Museux N, et al. Influence of thermal drive on central sleep apnea in the preterm neonate. Sleep 2008;31(4):549–56.

63. Khan A, Qurashi M, Kwiatkowski K, et al. Measurement of the CO_2 apneic threshold in newborn infants: possible relevance for periodic

breathing and apnea. J Appl Physiol 2005;98(4): 1171–6.

64. Vergales BD, Paget-Brown AO, Lee H, et al. Accurate automated apnea analysis in preterm infants. Am J Perinatol 2013. [Epub ahead of print].

65. Amin SB, Burnell E. Monitoring apnea of prematurity: validity of nursing documentation and bedside cardiorespiratory monitor. Am J Perinatol 2013; 30(8):643–8.

66. McGrath-Morrow SA, Ryan T, McGinley BM, et al. Polysomnography in preterm infants and children with chronic lung disease. Pediatr Pulmonol 2012; 47(2):172–9.

67. Das S, Mindell J, Millet GC, et al. Pediatric polysomnography: the patient and family perspective. J Clin Sleep Med 2011;7(1):81–7.

68. Kahlke PE, Witmans MB, Alabdoulsalam T, et al. Full-night versus 4h evening polysomnography in children less than 2 years of age. Sleep Med 2013;14(2):177–82.

69. Marcus CL, Keens TG, Ward SL. Comparison of nap and overnight polysomnography in children. Pediatr Pulmonol 1992;13(1):16–21.

70. Kirk VG, Bohn SG, Flemons WW, et al. Comparison of home oximetry monitoring with laboratory polysomnography in children. Chest 2003;124(5):1702–8.

71. Foo JY, Parsley CL, Wilson SJ, et al. Detection of central respiratory events using pulse transit time in infants. Conf Proc IEEE Eng Med Biol Soc 2005;3:2579–82.

72. Weintraub Z, Alvaro R, Kwiatkowski K, et al. Effects of inhaled oxygen (up to 40%) on periodic breathing and apnea in preterm infants. J Appl Physiol 1992;72(1):116–20.

73. Henderson-Smart DJ, Steer PA. Caffeine versus theophylline for apnea in preterm infants. Cochrane Database Syst Rev 2010;(1):CD000273.

74. Schmidt B, Roberts RS, Davis P, et al. Caffeine therapy for apnea of prematurity. N Engl J Med 2006;354(20):2112–21.

75. Schmidt B, Roberts RS, Davis P, et al. Long-term effects of caffeine therapy for apnea of prematurity. N Engl J Med 2007;357(19):1893–902.

76. Finer NN, Higgins R, Kattwinkel J, et al. Summary proceedings from the apnea-of-prematurity group. Pediatrics 2006;117(3 Pt 2):S47–51.

77. Bhat RY, Hannam S, Pressler R, et al. Effect of prone and supine position on sleep, apneas, and arousal in preterm infants. Pediatrics 2006;118(1): 101–7.

78. Alvaro RE, Khalil M, Qurashi M, et al. CO_2 inhalation as a treatment for apnea of prematurity: a randomized double-blind controlled trial. J Pediatr 2012;160(2):252–7.e1.

79. Al-Saif S, Alvaro R, Manfreda J, et al. A randomized controlled trial of theophylline versus CO_2 inhalation for treating apnea of prematurity. J Pediatr 2008;153(4):513–8.

80. Edwards BA, Sands SA, Feeney C, et al. Continuous positive airway pressure reduces loop gain and resolves periodic central apneas in the lamb. Respir Physiol Neurobiol 2009;168(3): 239–49.

81. Bloch-Salisbury E, Indic P, Bednarek F, et al. Stabilizing immature breathing patterns of preterm infants using stochastic mechanosensory stimulation. J Appl Physiol 2009;107(4): 1017–27.

82. Philippi H, Bieber I, Reitter B. Acetazolamide treatment for infantile central sleep apnea. J Child Neurol 2001;16(8):600–3.

83. Zagol K, Lake DE, Vergales B, et al. Anemia, apnea of prematurity, and blood transfusions. J Pediatr 2012;161(3):417–21.e1.

Index

Note: Page numbers of article titles are in **boldface** type.

A

Acetazolamide, for central sleep apnea and cardiovascular disease, 32
  for primary central sleep apnea, 3
Achondroplasia, central hypoventilation syndromes due to, 112–113
Acromegaly, central sleep apnea due to, 61
Adaptive servoventilation, in central sleep apnea, **69–85**
  alternatives to, 80
  devices and algorithms, 70–76
  effect on daytime symptoms and quality of life, 80
  efficacy according to severity of breathing disorder or underlying cardiac disease, 79–80
  for complex CSA syndrome, 42–44
  for CSA and cardiovascular disease, 31
  for CSA due to Cheyne-Stokes breathing pattern, 5
  in complex sleep apnea and other central disturbances, 81
  in heart failure patients, open questions on, 80–81
  in opioid-induced sleep apnea, 81–82
  influence on physiologic parameters and sympathoadrenergic activity, 79
  influence on respiratory disturbances and cardiovascular parameters, 77–79
  pathophysiologic background, 70
  titration and setting, 76–77
American Academy of Sleep Medicine (AASM), practice parameters for central sleep apnea, **1–11**
  caused by a drug or substance, 7
  caused by medical conditions other than Cheyne-Stokes, 7
  due to Cheyne-Stokes breathing pattern, 3–6
  due to high-altitude periodic breathing, 6–7
  primary, 2–3
Amyotrophic lateral sclerosis, central sleep apnea due 64, 63
Apnea. *See* Central sleep apnea.
Atrial fibrillation, and central sleep apnea, 32
Atrophy, multiple-system, central sleep apnea due to, 62
Autonomic dysregulation, rapid-onset obesity with hypothalamic dysfunction, hypoventilation, and, 110–111

B

Bilevel positive airway pressure (BPAP), for central sleep apnea due to Cheyne-Stokes breathing pattern, 5
  for complex CSA syndrome, 42
Body position, manipulation of, as alternate treatment for central sleep apnea, 101
Brain tumors, central sleep apnea due to, 60
Breathing, central control of, 58
  changes in inputs to, from wakefulness to sleep, 58–59
  normal control of, 105–107
Buprenorphine, opioid-induced central sleep apnea, **49–56**

C

Carbon dioxide, minimization of hypocapnia for central sleep apnea treatment, 89–94
Carbonic anhydrase inhibition, as alternate treatment for central sleep apnea, 97–98
Cardiac interventions, for central sleep apnea due to Cheyne-Stokes breathing pattern, 6
Cardiac pacing, for central sleep apnea in cardiovascular disease, 29
Cardiovascular disease, and central sleep apnea, **27–35**
  clinical implications of CSA in heart failure, 28–29
  epidemiology, 27–28
    of CSA in heart failure, 27–28
    of heart failure, 27
  treatment, 29–32
    novel drug therapy, 32
    pharmacologic intervention, 29
    positive airway pressure, 29–32
    surgery, devices, and cardiac pacing, 29
Central hypoventilation syndromes, achondroplasia, 112–113
  acquired conditions causing, 113
  Chiari malformation, 111–112
  congenital, 107–110
  familial dysautonomia, 111
  management of, 113–114
    diaphragmatic pacing, 114
    general considerations, 114
    negative pressure ventilation, 114
    positive pressure ventilation, 113–114

Moving?

Make sure your subscription moves with you!

To notify us of your new address, find your **Clinics Account Number** (located on your mailing label above your name), and contact customer service at:

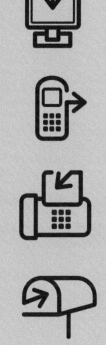

Email: journalscustomerservice-usa@elsevier.com

800-654-2452 (subscribers in the U.S. & Canada)
314-447-8871 (subscribers outside of the U.S. & Canada)

Fax number: 314-447-8029

Elsevier Health Sciences Division
Subscription Customer Service
3251 Riverport Lane
Maryland Heights, MO 63043

ELSEVIER

Printed and bound by CPI Group (UK) Ltd, Croydon, CR0 4YY

03/10/2024

01040381-0011